LIFE 2.0

Bala Shankar is an entrepreneur and writer based in Singapore. Bala has an MBA degree from the prestigious Indian Institute of Management, Ahmedabad, and had extended careers in corporate, consulting and university teaching in India, Singapore and the US. Bala worked in various sales, account management and leadership capacities for national and multinational companies. As an adjunct faculty, he was associated with teaching and executive education programmes at leading universities in Singapore. He is a contributor to *The Business Times*, Singapore, on various business and general topics. Bala published a B2B sales book, *Nuanced Account Management: Driving Excellence in B2B Sales*, in 2018 and a book on habits for skill-building, *The Twelve Habits of Smart Skill-Building: A Code for the Reskilling of You*, in 2021. He co-manages a K-12 institution that he co-founded in Singapore. Bala is a lover, writer and critic of Indian classical music. Writing is more than a hobby for Bala now, with a few works in the pipeline.

Praise for the Book

This is a creative, timely and valuable book for all adults. It invites us to move from Life 1.0 to Life 2.0; from a life primarily for self and family, to one for society also. It is a call for PSR—Personal Social Responsibility. It gives examples of people who have moved on to Life 2.0, and created legacies which will outlast them. The book shows how you can do it. It is our dharma and duty to do so.

—**Dr Mrityunjay B. Athreya**, DBA (Harvard), Padma Bhushan awardee, management advisor and author

We have only one life, and most of us examine it only once—towards the end—unless a life-threatening moment forces an examination. Bala's *Life 2.0* provides the opportunity to reflect upon life early on, without an accident! The 12 mandates are powerful triggers that are bound to set you on a new and more meaningful course in your life.

—**Rajendra S. Pawar**, Padma Bhushan awardee, co-founder and chairman, NIIT Ltd.

I found *Life 2.0* to be a thoughtful book, rooted in rich personal experiences told with simplicity and authenticity. Take it with you on a weekend retreat...accept its invitation and nudge to reflect on your life and think about how you want to live the rest of it...you will come back enriched and renewed.

—**Professor Rama Bijapurkar**, professor, Indian Institute of Management, Ahmedabad, thought leader and independent board director

Many of us have gone through times when we start to seek a reset on many matters concerning our lives. Bala Shankar has presented a compelling idea that such opportunities should be used to plan and do things that could shape our legacy. As his gentle narrative in *Life 2.0* comes with memorable anecdotes, readers will surely find the various ideas highly relevant and practical.

—**Professor Rajendra Srivastava**, MBA and PhD,
Former dean, Indian School of Business (ISB) and
Novartis Professor of Marketing Strategy and Innovation

As our life expectancy is growing, the number of productive years post-retirement is substantial. Merely waiting for that moment is not ideal. This book is a great way for those in their forties and fifties, to start planning and building a meaningful legacy that will positively impact and drive the second phase of life.

—**Meena Ganesh**, MBA, Co-founder, MD and CEO,
Portea Medical. Entrepreneur and
former promoter of TruVista

LIFE 2.0
YOUR BEST CHANCE TO SCRIPT YOUR LEGACY

Bala Shankar

Published by
Rupa Publications India Pvt. Ltd 2022
7/16, Ansari Road, Daryaganj
New Delhi 110002

Sales centres:
Allahabad Bengaluru Chennai
Hyderabad Jaipur Kathmandu
Kolkata Mumbai

Copyright © Bala Shankar 2022

The views and opinions expressed in this book are the
authors' own and the facts are as reported by him which
have been verified to the extent possible, and the publishers
are not in any way liable for the same.

All rights reserved.
No part of this publication may be reproduced, transmitted,
or stored in a retrieval system, in any form or by any means,
electronic, mechanical, photocopying, recording or otherwise,
without the prior permission of the publisher.

ISBN: 978-93-5520-405-9

First impression 2022

10 9 8 7 6 5 4 3 2 1

The moral right of the author has been asserted.

Printed in India

This book is sold subject to the condition that it shall not,
by way of trade or otherwise, be lent, resold, hired out, or otherwise
circulated, without the publisher's prior consent, in any form of
binding or cover other than that in which it is published.

To the health and frontline workers who risked their lives to care for the affected people during the COVID-19 pandemic.

A part of the author's estimated income from this publication has been donated for their welfare.

CONTENTS

Foreword — xi
Preface — xiii
Introduction — xv

1. The Mandates: Coordinates of a New Journey — 1
   - Learning New Skills — 4
   - Impacting Society — 22
   - Revisiting Missed Opportunities — 38
   - Reassessing Goals — 49
   - Decoupling Finances and Life — 64
   - Being Grateful and Gracious — 81
   - Sharing and Coaching — 97
   - Reshaping Communication — 113
   - Working without Rewards — 128
   - Acquiring Social Assets — 140
   - Being Ourselves — 155
   - Moderating the Ego — 166

2.	The Story of How My Life 2.0 Began...	178
3.	The Beginning	188

Acknowledgements   191

FOREWORD

For over two decades of my career as a cricket player, captain, coach and administrator, I was fortunate to be a part of the centre stage both in India and abroad. Apart from the enjoyment of playing a popular sport, I was blessed with achievements, records and honours that I am certainly proud of. However, I have always pondered on what I want to be known for. This is a stock question in interviews as well. I am convinced that it has to go beyond my cricket story. This book by Bala Shankar addresses this issue from many interesting angles. It expands on the concept of living life in a number of purposeful ways, all of which help develop a good personal story at all times. Everybody secretly wishes for a good legacy, and I am sure that the readers will find the hand-holding style of narration useful, pertinent and an important call to action.

—**Anil Kumble**, former Indian cricketer, captain and coach; former chair, Cricket Council of the International Cricket Council; record holder for the most test and one-day international wickets for India

PREFACE

You are in your forties, fifties or sixties and have seen a lot of water flow under the bridge of life. Your life has been full of major and minor events. Perhaps you are riding a wave of success and happiness, or you have had better days. Your life may be running mechanically or you may have managed to spice it up with meaningful variety. You believe that you have most matters under control or you are annoyed that you are not able to shape everything the way you would like to. Either way, you are still active, productive, engaged, resourceful and interested in enriching your life. Here is an anecdotal maxim: you are not any different from 99 per cent of the people on this planet with respect to any of these situations. Life, however, is more than all these aspects. Life is a great opportunity, even if it remains a challenge. Life is the result of all the choices that we make or are made for us. How can our lives, therefore, become an active tool in our hands? What introspection, planning and steering will help us do this? What would we want to do if we get the right to script the remainder of our lives and, indeed, our legacies? These are perfect questions to ask. They are also the premise of this book and the stimuli for our discussion.

INTRODUCTION

Life is a singular word. The general sense is that it is one unit—from birth to death—and when we refer to life, we mean the period in between. In reality, however, life is a sum of many parts, phases, scenes and events. It moves from one phase to another, one physical place to another, one state of mind to another, one accomplishment or failure to another, one experience to another, one set of interests and pursuits to others and one circle of people to another. Thus, one life is a composite of many sub-lives. Sometimes, we talk of having received a new lease of life, especially when we recover from illnesses or near-fatal encounters. This alludes to physical survival (and rebirth, if you will). However, in one's life, there are moments when things seem to be changing a tad too much—some disruptive changes, some about-turns, some courses that we orchestrate and some that seem orchestrated for us. All of these moments of change can be considered tipping points. Many of you would have experienced such points at least once. The more dramatic the change caused by this tipping point, the more it looks like a new life. So, our lives stop and restart at several points. Therefore, I prefer to call each of these tipping points as the start of Life 2.0, 3.0, and so on.

Mahatma Gandhi who was born in India but lived away from his country for decades returned to India from South Africa at the age of 45 to participate in the struggle for freedom from British colonial rule alongside his people. His legacy is now built around his life thereafter. Abraham Lincoln joined the Republican Party around the age of 45, and before he turned 60, he had become the iconic president of his country and died in office. His handling of the American Civil War is now a significant moment in American history. His legacy flows directly from those tumultuous years during which he left his mark. Considered to be one of the founders and the father of modern-day Carnatic music, Purandara Dasa lived in the sixteenth century.[1] He was a diamond merchant who inherited enormous wealth from his family business. He multiplied it further and was even considered a miser. Some time in his forties, he switched professions and became an ardent admirer and worshipper of Lord Vishnu (considered the protector in the Hindu trilogy of gods). He also started writing and structuring Carnatic music, especially as a learner's text. Nearly 500 years later, his structure for Carnatic music is still in vogue.

What do all the people discussed above have in common? These people, and many others like them, encountered a life-changing event later in their lives and led a Life 2.0

---

[1]Sri Purandara Dasa Memorial Trust, https://tinyurl.com/z8p5m99j.

that was very different from their lives before—one that set up their enduring legacies. Gandhi and Lincoln are not famous for their legal practices, and Purandara Dasa is not a legend of the diamond trade. So, what can we learn from their lives? For one, they embraced Life 2.0 with open arms when it called them. They also lived the perfect Life 2.0 that shaped their legacies.

Perhaps not everyone would encounter such a radical change in their lives. Nonetheless, everyone does get opportunities to engineer the shifts in his or her life. Even if it is not about building a famous legacy, we all silently harbour the need to be well-regarded and praised for the right reasons when we are gone. This legacy motivator underpins most of the concepts in this book.

My motivation to write this book came from a similar crossroad in my life. I experienced such a turn of events in 2006 (briefly shared in the penultimate chapter, see page 178), and have christened my life since then as Life 2.0. More than 15 years later, I have reflected on my Life 2.0 and attempted to characterize the changes and their aftermath, the lessons I learned along the way and my new efforts and their early results. It became increasingly clear to me that my current life was not the same as my Life 1.0, and that shift had major implications for the way I saw and understood my new life, embraced it and got around to living it...differently. I am not running a legacy-making project. But I have some hopes that when my Life 2.0 ends, I would have left enough behind to add up to a legacy. I certainly don't consider my story unique. It is a story of one human being. Yet, the lessons or mandates that I postulate in this book may offer a pattern that others could expect or may have seen around in their lives. This book aims to reflect on this fascinating journey with some sense of reasoning and comprehension—a connection that our rational minds crave.

When this book reaches your hands, our generation would have endured the worst pandemic in over a century that stalled a lot of lives, took some, realigned many and brought others to a crossroad in search of new directions. Through the COVID-19 pandemic, humanity faced a Life 2.0 situation, and some are still relaunching their disrupted lives. Amid this havoc, the human spirit has responded to the call of duty admirably. It promises to lead us to Life 2.0 with undeterred hopes, this time, with our own design. This Life 2.0 moment, thus, needs a coach. While I don't promise to be that coach, I hope to be a speaking partner through this book.

Peer-to-peer Angle

The field of self-improvement is littered with books and lectures that predominantly talk 'to' the reader or the listener. It is an unequal relationship between the writer or the speaker and their audience. It is not a level playing field, as the former is supposed to be more learned, evolved or competent. Such learning tools have the unmistakable sense of being sermons. As a contrast, I want this book to be a peer-to-peer journey of reading and reflection where I am talking 'with' you (as you read the book, I imagine you nodding). Therefore, I would want this to be our shared journey. Let us try to grasp the phenomenon of a life transition together.

If someone asked you, 'What's your life's report card?' How would you respond? Is it made up of just one or two facets like money, career, education, power or position? We forget to talk about many other things that we may have embraced or ignored. Like a school report card, what grades would you give yourself for each subject or module of your lives, or for the aspects of lives that we may have neglected? Asked about her journey, a diplomat at the United Nations said, 'People always want me to talk about what I do and not what I am. It's that oft-asked question that set me to reflect on what I am.'

Change is a Given

Life is a great big canvas; throw all the paint you can at it.

—Danny Kaye

Our lives can change in two ways. One is gradual and the other is a more sudden shift, like the COVID-19 pandemic. When Life 1.0 changes gradually, many small and big changes keep happening at different points, although these may not be cataclysmic or discontinuous. For example, changes to marriage, partner and family are typical. Other forms of gradual and normative changes include changing jobs or moving to another place. These happen at regular intervals and have a seamless pattern. In some ways, these are linear changes that occur with some predictability to their sequence and timing. Since these changes occur somewhat mechanically, we are able to embrace them subconsciously and go with the flow. This is not to suggest that there is no thought behind these shifts. Our thinking about these changes centres on choices, directions and timing. However, we tend to reflect less on saying 'yes' or 'no' to these shifts. For example, few people deliberately opt to not marry or work for a living, and most people carefully consider their decisions about 'who' they want to marry or what profession or job they want to pursue. There is an air of inevitability to these processes and their sequence. It almost suggests to us that such gradual changes are pre-destined, and as long as they are normative, our minds and bodies are willing and equipped to embrace them. We even seek them because we want to be normal.

Is life meant to be mechanical and largely auto-piloted? No. There is often a new angle to life brought in by the more disruptive nature of changes, which can be sudden, shocking, unsettling and profound. By nature, these changes would normally be externally induced and storm in without notice. The COVID-19 pandemic checks all the boxes for being an external disruptive change. In some rare cases, people seem to embrace sudden changes, but in reality, they must have thought about these changes for a long time before embracing them—someone leaving the family life to seek sainthood, for example. Disruptive occurrences are infrequent (they may happen once or twice in one's life) and can potentially affect a number of areas in our lives—income, family, location, career, relationships, attitudes, passion, etc. They have the power to turn our lives topsy-turvy with either damaging or positive consequences. In some cases, they could also be initiated from within. For example, a natural calamity or the loss of a loved one could be external factors that force some realignment. Reflections, introspection, a new spiritual thought or mentor could be sources of disruptive change that come from within. The circumstances that lead to both types of disruptive changes could have some common threads. The loss of a beloved family member may awaken the inner self and give rise to new thoughts. These may culminate in decisions that have a far-reaching impact on our lives and on the lives of people around us. For instance, the Indian emperor Ashoka embraced Buddhism and non-violence after being distraught at the sight of dead bodies after the Kalinga war that he started and won. Therefore, it can be said that this external event triggered his transformation. People may switch suddenly from a professional career to politics. That is usually the result of an internal thought process. Thus, it is important to understand the two types of changes and their distinctive nature and sources to be able to start thinking of Life 2.0. Irrespective of the triggers and their sources, Life 2.0 has the propensity to change our résumé, often distinctively. Thus, it is a legacy-making moment.

Longer Life and a New Reset

*Everyone thinks of changing the world,
but no one thinks of changing himself.*

—Leo Tolstoy

The concept of Life 2.0 could be seen as a necessity. Humans are living longer now. In most advanced economies and even in less developed nations, urban life expectancy is 75 years or more. With 20–30 years in our sunset years, we need new experiences, tools and, of course, talents and skills to not meander. Our sunset years are no longer meant to pull down the shutters and wait for the inevitable end. Living healthily until 75–80 forces us to reflect on shaping our Life 2.0. More wealth, comfort and reminiscing of the past glory are not going to do this for us. A reset of the self-will to rediscover life in new ways beckons us and calls for action. One could view this concept as an amalgamation of two lives—one that we live and the other that we leave behind (our legacy). It is not necessary that we embark on changes only when we sink to the bottom, one way or the other. In fact, a seamless, proactive migration into Life 2.0 is even more commendable than when it is done in response to a cataclysmic event.

INTRODUCTION

Our early lives are largely influenced by our parents, immediate friends, relatives and people who we meet in schools, colleges, workplaces, our local environment, etc. The safe option is to remain in the general mainstream and do what most people did. This normative behaviour covers our education, sports, recreational pursuits, clothing, food, language, habits, entertainment and even style. As we grow up, our marriage, career and family choices are also shaped by our social contexts. This is even truer of Asian and other conservative societies. For example, in my generation, we could count on one hand the number of inter-religious marriages or off-beat careers—like owning or operating a restaurant, photography, linguistics or painting—in our family circles. With every subsequent generation, these numbers have grown, and norm-breaking behaviours are more common today. It would be more appropriate to say that new norms are being set.

As a person born in the baby boomer era, my attitudes were very much conformist too. I followed the conventional wisdom of acquiring many degrees as soon as possible, marrying, having children, pursuing a successful career, etc. However, my life wasn't entirely predictable. I managed to introduce some interesting twists along the way.

By and large, this seemed like my Life 1.0, since its patterns were linear, and changes were incremental and largely logical. There were no major upheavals and an astrologically minded person would call it the reign of Jupiter—a long one at that! I was lucky to progress well in a career that presented me with global responsibilities, gave me a steady rise in income and took me to the great new city of Singapore. I also had a happy family and got to watch my dear daughter grow into a confident young adolescent, ready to go to college. Then things started to happen…

In 2006, everything in my life seemed to change. These changes came so dramatically and quickly that I didn't have the time to absorb them fully. Suffice to say, I was in the midst of a life storm, which I didn't decode well until much later.

Coincidentally, my mind was on a path of exploration, search, learning, unlearning, assimilation and reflection at the same time. I was seeking new directions, pursuits and experiences. Such moments occur in all our lives, perhaps a few times. I was fortunate that I could think about the many aspects of my life, not just my career and finances. In fact, finances were among my smaller concerns. My wife and I took small steps to downsize our needs (for instance, we went car-less for four years) and assess our ability to come to terms with them. We managed to sail through that phase and were lucky to build the mental strength to be able to adapt to any lifestyle. The series of thoughts triggered during this phase led me to various pursuits—some, immediately and others, later. These formed the script of my Life 2.0.

If anyone reaches a point where life seems to take a turn into versions 2.0 or 3.0, these patterns could be valuable guides. At least they would offer insights that you perhaps find common cause with. I don't promise any new revelations but some rational cues from a person who has been there and done that. I hope this book serves another simple purpose. When we try to engineer a change in our lives or attitudes, we become seekers. Those who preach or guide the seekers seem to be out of the ordinary, like spiritual gurus, magicians, cult or mass movement leaders, etc. By all accounts, I belong to none of these categories. I am one of you, and all I intend to do is offer lateral guidance and conversation.

The Twelve Mandates

The 12 mandates that I describe in this book became beacons guiding my Life 2.0. In many of these postulates, I am more at their introductory stage, with a lot more potential ground to cover. In many ways, these mandates have the potential to make up my story, more than my accomplishments in Life 1.0. I hope that you would feel the same about launching your own Life 2.0.

We are in the midst of a big debate about success and happiness, and how one does not guarantee the other. This book is not about how to succeed. It is also not about how to be happy. It is about how we can engineer our lives and actions at a certain point in life so that we sow the seeds to be remembered well, and to define the code for our legacy.

This book does not intend to make its readers feel guilty either. What you did in Life 1.0 is history. It happened under certain circumstances, in a certain state of mind and for certain priorities that were relevant at those points of time. I would want this book to be read without any remorse about the past and purely as a map for the future, without demanding any confessions. Thus, we begin with a clean slate. Without any past baggage, let us take forward only the learnings and maturity that our past affords us.

In this context, it is useful to realize and accept that we will neither be able to change everything about or around us nor what we go through. Life 1.0 spreads some moss on our personality that will be difficult to remove. Similarly, our family, surroundings and circumstances are a given and cannot be changed significantly. So, without seeking to change what we cannot, we should have a desire to set in motion a personal evolution programme that moulds the circumstances that can be changed and are reasonably in our control (unless you fancy yourself to be the next Gandhi, Lincoln or Purandara Dasa).

This is the genesis of this book. The mandates, which are more of gentle self-mandates, will hopefully get you thinking on these lines in a structured manner. Each mandate has been elaborated on in the subsequent sections of this book, providing the meaning, scope and anecdotal support that would define it more clearly. More importantly, I have tried to postulate why they are relevant and how they could benefit us. The beauty of these mandates is that one could embrace them without feeling any pressure or undue guilt of not having tried them so far. They are not meant to substitute our current life patterns but to co-exist with them, gradually forming new decisive patterns in our lives. Hopefully, they will also lead to a better sense of fulfilment, even if it is unquantifiable.

Let me also declare that I have generally tried to avoid religious or spiritual references while dealing with the mandates. Texts like the Bhagavad Gita (the sacred text of the Hindus) have been cited in a couple of places as a neutral reference. Thus, I have maintained a practical character in the narration. For want of a better word, this book has an irreligious tone. I have used the terms mandates, commandments and postulates interchangeably.

Finally, the narrative carefully avoids taking an altruistic tone since I want the ideas in the book to be understandable and applicable for everyone. It is not a guru's perspective. Even if you are not the type wishing for a lasting legacy or an entirely new life, these ideas will guide you towards a life that is entirely scripted by you from now on, and for those who need a post-pandemic reset, it will offer a new thought process.

THE MANDATES: COORDINATES OF A NEW JOURNEY

All new journeys need coordinates (even the GPS needs it). When we gear up for a new life journey, it may not necessarily start with a big bang or by turning on a switch. Life is a dial. There is no clear end to Life 1.0 and beginning for Life 2.0. It could be a seamless transition or, in some sense, a continuation of some things that germinated in your Life 1.0. So, there is newness to Life 2.0, but there is also continuity. Everything is not rejigged. Thus, the reference to Life 2.0 is more spatial and symbolic than time-determined.

Our larger interests will be the consequences of the legacy-rich activities that I propose in this book. I do bring my own experiences and anecdotes from my Life 2.0 as evidence across the book, but I do not dwell on the moments that triggered my shifts, since they are not important and may wade into my life story, which is not the purpose of this book.

All good beginnings are sometimes plagued by doubts—beware of them. In today's social-media-driven world, pros and cons of every hypothesis are advocated relentlessly, landing directly into your inboxes. They sometimes lead to doubts, which slow you down or could even make you abandon the good steps you have taken. Therefore, you need a crusade of sorts to carry these out consistently. Get into a dogged mindset and don't slacken your pace due to intellectual paralysis. The good thing is that you can attempt the mandates in the book in small measures, and the tide of progress will take you further. Even more comforting is the fact that none of the mandates have any downsides—you have everything to gain and nothing to lose! So, be a resolute warrior!

Assuming that you are keen to explore rebooting your life, or you feel that it already has a new direction, here are my 12 mandates to guide you into Life 2.0:

1. Learning new skills
2. Impacting society
3. Revisiting missed opportunities
4. Reassessing goals
5. Decoupling finances and life
6. Being grateful and gracious
7. Sharing and coaching
8. Reshaping communication
9. Working without rewards
10. Acquiring social assets
11. Being ourselves
12. Moderating the ego

THE MANDATES: COORDINATES OF A NEW JOURNEY

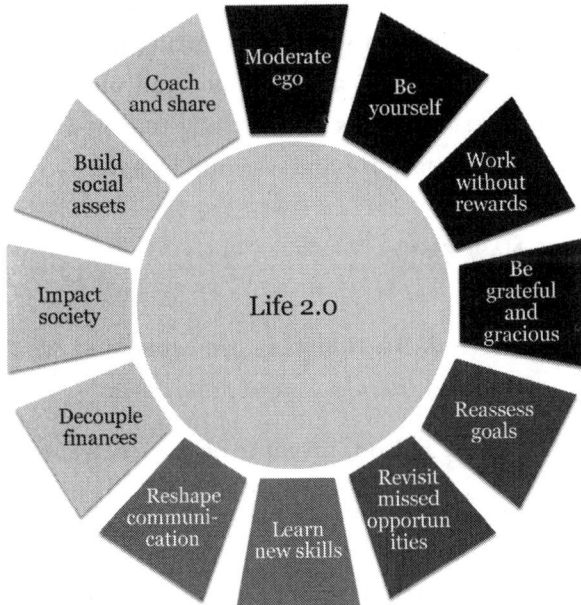

These mandates can be taken up one after another, simultaneously or in clusters. We need to take the lead to implement these mandates, as there is no external motivating force.

You would also recognize that some of these are inter-related, although, at a conceptual level, we can study them separately. Life is an amalgam of all its elements, and Life 2.0 is no different. In fact, the inter-connectedness lends itself well for us to exploit our multiple facets.

Your journey with the book would also instigate you towards 'self-awareness', a highly sought-after trait among leaders, which is evangelized by many modern authors in management. You pivot the transformation, and, therefore, your assessment of yourself is the starting point.

I hope I have motivated you to read about what to expect during the process of switching to a new life—Life 2.0—with a new purpose and a proud legacy.

Learning New Skills

> *If we did all the things we are capable of, we would literally astound ourselves.*

—Thomas A. Edison, inventor of the electric bulb

In a matter of about 10 years, many of our old capabilities have been questioned, especially in the workplace. There is a clarion call from all quarters to reskill ourselves for the future. This is not only to enable us to earn or maintain our livelihood but also to move with the times, as technology encompasses every aspect of our lives. The Singapore government, for instance, has a whole new ministry ('skillsfuture'[1]) set up to identify and drive the acquisition of new work skills for the entire population. In this section, we examine skills that could complement our professional capabilities or develop our faculties better while sharpening our life-long learning aptitude. Even if it is not a vocational need for some of us, revitalizing our ability to learn new things is one of the keys to Life 2.0.

---

[1] SkillsFuture, https://tinyurl.com/mfntuc83. Accessed on 4 April 2022.

THE MANDATES: COORDINATES OF A NEW JOURNEY

There is no better place to begin our journey to reboot our lives than ourselves—specifically what we are capable of. Yes, we are a lot more capable than we settle for. We have defined our limits by not exploring further. A major part of our skill acquisition happens when we are young, especially before we turn 30. It's not just numeracy, literacy and logic, but other trainable skills like typing, driving, basic computer skills, mechanical skills, music, art, sports, etc. Communication and social skills are also picked up from the environment that we are exposed to, and by modelling ourselves on the people around us. Our levels of competency in each skill may vary, and often, our skill levels hover around 4–8 on a scale of 10 (10 being outstanding). The problem is, we are not aware of these levels, and no one really measures them. The learning quietly stops once the skill levels reach a deployable scale (in some instances, even before that).

The period after reaching this skill level suddenly becomes barren in terms of furthering the skill. Subsequently, we apply our available skills and start a career. In fact, it even seems that we have reached the end of our formal skill pursuit. We are lulled into believing that new skills are not necessary for our career or life, as most things seem to be going smoothly and in tune with our intentions. This is the result of the tapering of incentives—financial, social or individual. Oddly, therefore, skills are identified as a means to achieve something rather than an end in themselves. Think of all the things that you started when you were young and didn't quite continue to a logical stage.

Skill-building is an important input to the kind of things that we want to do after a certain point—in Life 2.0. In a very connected way, new skills combine with old ones and propel us into areas where we can participate well. Our footprint in such areas flows into the legacy jigsaw. Mahatma Gandhi found that his patience and persuasion skills paved the way for his epoch-making achievement of leading the Indian liberation movement as opposed to the argumentative streak that he perhaps picked up from his legal profession. New pursuits need new skills (and new skills lead to new pursuits). Understanding that our skillsets need to evolve or be replaced is, thus, a core theme of Life 2.0.

Have any of you ever felt awkward that you can't make a good cup of tea, sew a button on a shirt, assemble your IKEA table or write a budget for a small family event that you are planning? Years pass by as we keep taking help to do all these things. We also think highly of other skills that seem to run our careers and lives. In a self-serving way, we tend to focus on our strengths and ignore our weaknesses. If you draw up a list of the various skills of an average person, you will perhaps see yourself being good at 25 per cent, or less, of that list. Please undertake this exercise and see what it reveals. We are not even cognizant of the limitations we place on ourselves. Changing times bring with them new skill sets that may even become absolutely necessary to acquire. The smartphone revolution, online transactions (especially flight or hotel bookings), operating self-service counters and kiosks are a few examples of how our survival

THE MANDATES: COORDINATES OF A NEW JOURNEY

kit can change profoundly. The COVID-19 pandemic added to the list of skills that are essential for survival—patience, self-help, adding a spark to family ties, working effectively online and a very different communication style. Several other areas that we may have ignored become useful at a later point in life (tying a bowtie can be a simple example). We also become curious about certain skills and want to put our mind to them (mountain climbing, for instance). As we see other people around us acquiring many new skills to navigate their daily lives, we become conscious of our shortcomings. Even at this point, there is a marked difference between knowing the gaps and doing something to address them. This is where learning a new skill becomes relevant. It nudges us to do something about our shortcomings.

Here, we must ask ourselves two questions—do we wait till our current skill sets are exhausted before seeking new ones? And how does the mind overcome inertia (or complacency) and drive us to acquire the next skill sets?

There are many people who do this early in life. Mark Zuckerberg, founder and CEO of Meta, is fluent in Mandarin and spoke to university students in China in their language.[2] Now, Zuckerberg is not likely to have had 'spare time' to learn one of the most difficult languages to master, amid his more important tasks of founding and running a rapidly growing company! He just did it.

---

[2]Taylor, Adam. 'Mark Zuckerberg gave a 20-minute speech in Mandarin to Chinese students', *The Washington Post*, 26 October 2015, https://tinyurl.com/42mv5253. Accessed on 4 April 2022.

For others, the window of Life 2.0 may spur them on to learn. Life 2.0 is an opportunity to revisit the settled notion of our skill-learnability. We realize, during the first phase of our career and life, that we lack many skills. Some may not be confident presenters, others may lack linguistic abilities, be poor at physical sports or writing, be introverts or procrastinators, find it difficult to make friends and so on. Some of these skill gaps may impact people's career or life prospects, thereby hastening the incentive to learn them. We do naturally acquire a few new skills while dealing with our professional and family lives.

However, some skills may not directly impact our careers, and may need more dedicated time and inclination from us. Life 2.0 offers us that luxury. Mahatma Gandhi said, 'Live as if you were to die tomorrow. Learn as if you were to live forever.' If you are willing to put aside the time and dogged effort required to learn, it can be done. It may not be rewarding in the traditional sense. However, the pride of acquiring a new skill at a later stage in life is unique and unexplainable. Many people from my generation had to learn to operate a computer, use the internet and technological tools like Microsoft Word, Excel, emails, online transactions, e-books, etc. While some worked tirelessly and managed to bridge the gap with the succeeding generations, others did not even try. I know of several people in their sixties and seventies who need secretaries to do any of these computer- and internet-related tasks. Some people still do not reply to emails themselves and others need help to operate even

THE MANDATES: COORDINATES OF A NEW JOURNEY

plug-and-play devices. So, there is a lot of inner resistance to overcome. Learning atrophy is an outcome many do not even recognize.

I embarked on acquiring a few skills at the onset of my Life 2.0. I was curious to learn more about my religion, Hinduism, its historic texts and meanings. I attended classes with a traditional priest to learn Hindu shlokas (prayer verses) including the powerful *Rudram and Chamakam* (shlokas on Lord Shiva) and *sooktham*s. It took me about a year to learn, recite from memory and polish my new skill—learning over 2,000 words in Sanskrit, which was a new language for me. These verses have both lyrics and a certain oscillating rhythm that must be perfectly rendered. As with any skill, one is likely to get habituated to it gradually, and this is likely to be even slower if you are not young. I had to practice my recitation regularly and with fanatic interest in order to overcome the slow pace of learning and absorption that sets in when you cross your forties. It may not be a simple skill to acquire and may not engage everyone, but the age makes it harder. The more traditional Hindu children learn this at the age of seven or eight and master it very quickly. To keep it fresh in your mind, you need to practice regularly after learning it. I recite these verses during my weekly prayers to Lord Shiva, which gives me the opportunity to practice them. It may sound less like a skill than knowledge, but the skill is in the acquisition and retention of a difficult text. This is more challenging, especially in a new language, and if it is solely dependent on the student, as was my case.

I also got interested in the critique of South Indian classical music—generally known as Carnatic music. Like Western music concert or movie critics, a Carnatic music critic attends live concerts and reviews or critiques them. The reviews published in popular English newspapers are read not only by the listeners but also by the artistes and organizers. So, a critic is supposed to have reached an acceptable level of understanding and taste in music, besides having the ability to articulate his thoughts about it. These were challenges I had to overcome.

I had intermittently learnt Carnatic vocal music during my adult years and had developed some skill to appreciate it. I am thankful for this early learning, even though I harboured no intention of achieving any level of mastery in those days. This underlines the point that many of the pursuits we take up when we are young can be revived in some way when we are older. To critically analyse performances and publish an analysis, new skills that bring to the fore a variety in style, language, emphasis, critical tone, etc., are required, even though no one teaches them. So, I put together a self-teaching programme that included extensively listening to music—over a 3-year period, I listened to about 1,500 hours of recorded music by different artistes—speaking to performers, reading up the literature on topics related to music, learning various writing styles, comparatively analysing different performers, etc. I had to teach myself to sing some songs to gain more knowledge about the composition styles, intricacies, difficulties and the inherent beauty of this genre of music. These efforts came to a head towards the end of 2006. In 2007, my first review was published in *The Hindu*, a newspaper which covers the grand, annual, two-month Chennai Music Season, touted to be among the largest music festivals in the world. This music and dance festival, also known as the Chennai Sangamam, has earned Chennai the United Nations Educational, Scientific and Cultural Organization (UNESCO) tag of a 'creative city' in 2017.[3] Since 2007, I have reviewed concerts at the Chennai Sangamam every year. I write and publish about 10 to 12 reviews, often waking up early to get my creative juices flowing. These reviews are read by both common readers and artistes. Therefore, they need to strike a fine balance between the readers' language and the artistes' lexicon—a blend of technical insights and consumerist analysis. As critics, we are also performers in some sense, aiming to get the approval of our readers. In the initial years, I would send the links to my reviews to friends and relatives, not just to seek a pat on the back (although it is always nice to have it) but to look for ways to improve, if anyone suggested them. As an extension of this skill, I offered to edit a book that was brought out to mark my grandfather's centenary, as he was also a Carnatic music critic. The ability to critique Carnatic music also led me to study its rich, 500–600-year-long history. Any history

---

[3] UNESCO Creative Cities Network, https://tinyurl.com/sndr2pbn. Accessed on 4 April 2022.

and its evolution is fascinating to me, and I have immensely enjoyed reading and understanding how an art form that was limited to artistes, royal courts and temples is now publicly performed, that too on a commercial scale. As with any skill, the more you practise it, the more you refine it, and I hope I am on this track. I consider this a proud achievement, as there is no formal way to learn this skill. There are also no clear benchmarks that I could aspire to. While I am satisfied with where I have reached, I am fully aware that there are many more peaks to climb.

The pursuit of these skills was triggered in me by new desires. Perhaps these had been latent in my system but manifested only later in life. My drive to acquire these skills must have been quite intense because I was able to persist with learning both and brought them to a fair conclusion. These are, by no means, path-breaking but that's also the beauty of this mandate on new skills. As long as it aligns with your desires, your effort is significant and the outcome is decent, it satisfies the mandate. Furthermore, these new skills can pivot us into new life-spaces, which may link us to our legacy.

We may start acquiring a new skill but may not be able to fulfil it. Some skills may take forever to acquire, and our efforts may lose steam. Just ask all the people who have carried a golf kit or a guitar in their car boots for years, without getting anywhere! There is also the proverbial 'valley of despair', a phase when your efforts and progress nosedive for various reasons. However, it is possible to pick up where you left off with a fresh dose of determination. I have had similar experiences too. The drive to reach the finishing line is determined by how satisfied you feel about possessing the skill or other self-esteem motives that may be latent. There may be no external recognition or monetary rewards, as in the two examples I mentioned in this section. In the theory propounded by Abraham Maslow,[4] the craving to acquire a new skill can be classified under self-esteem and perhaps even self-actualization needs. Progress monitoring and assessments for acquiring new skills should be an internal measure. The degree to which you master the skill is difficult to define and may never be known since fluency is only one aspect of mastery. In some ways, the challenge of self-learning and setting your own milestones brings further joy to these pursuits.

Young learners vs old learners

It is interesting to study the differences in the learning patterns between young and old people. One of the main differences is the source of learning. As an adult, it is sometimes difficult for us to accept that we cannot self-teach everything and that we may need a tutor. We tend to assume that our cerebral capacity has matured enough to follow instructions. In such cases, even if we manage to acquire a skill, the process is not time- or cost-efficient. For

---

[4] McLeod, Saul. 'Maslow's Hierarchy of Needs', SimplyPsychology, 2007, https://tinyurl.com/y2buhbfn. Accessed on 4 April 2022.

example, technically, you could pick up simple yoga skills by watching myriad YouTube lessons. However, many of these skills involve some dos and don'ts that may need a guru to make us learn and understand better. The other difference is in the duration of learning. One of my bosses was learning to play golf for about 10 years! He had the full kit loaded in his boot all the time. His poor practice frequency, lack of routine, low priority for the lesson and the absence of a burning desire to learn kept him away from real progress. Perhaps he was conscious of his rate of learning, so he did not see the light at the end of the tunnel. More likely, however, is the possibility that he, like most adults, threw in the towel too soon. On the contrary, young learners are more determined to pass any test to acquire a skill. They are also capable of calibrating their efforts to keep up with the required pace. These crucial aspects desert us as we grow older.

Young learners are more likely to approach their learning solo. Their minds are curious and patient (with a lot less ego), and their bodies are able and flexible. Thus, several trials and errors are acceptable to them as long as they see themselves progressing over time. As adult learners, we are often better off in company. A group setting is more conducive to our motivation and competitive instinct. We tend to find role models in our own group. These impact our rate and manner of learning. Group learning as a technique is even more useful if the skill-acquisition process is long and has several milestones.

For most young people, acquiring new skills may make the difference between leading a good life or a difficult one. They seek to master languages, a sport or a routine to improve the chances of succeeding at college or work. This motivation is lesser for adults, who are likely to be pursuing something for its own sake.

Learning is not followed by a full stop. An adult's learning pursuits need not be tethered to professional outcomes. This is both good and bad. Good because it can follow its own parallel patient track; but it is also bad because it is likely to be left halfway at any point of time.

One of the recommended adult learning techniques is viewing the process as a staircase or a set of staircases with several landings. We move a step at a time and we pause at the landings (intermediate milestones). We catch our breath again to walk up to the next landing. We do not have the option of staying on a step for long. In order to make our skill acquisition cumulative, we could visualize this analogy whenever our will becomes weak.

Why acquire a new skill?

Let us review some of the known and subtle benefits of acquiring a new skill. Besides enabling us to perform that new skill as a hobby or as part of our profession, acquiring a new skill impacts our physiology in many ways that we don't even know. It aids the formation of a higher number of connections between neurons, which helps us learn more and retain more information. As such connections get stronger, we have to think less about what we're doing (as these skills move into auto mode), which means we can get better at other facets of a set of skills. Think of how we drive a car once we ace it as opposed to our driving skill during our initial lessons. It has also been proven in a study done at the University of Texas at Austin that the brain expands every time it learns something.[5] The process of learning, which includes reading, watching, absorbing, checking, understanding, repeating, retaining, recalling, etc., is known to raise the brain activity and slow down the onset of afflictions like dementia, as brain cells come into play during any learning. One of my uncles, who developed dementia and lost his battle to it, could play all his songs on the harmonica till the very end but could not recognize people!

Once we learn a new skill, it can be a source of elation similar to how we feel when we conquer something. New skills will also lead us to new groups of people and social renewal. For instance, if you acquire cooking skills beyond a passable level, you will get the opportunity to be in the midst of chefs, ingredient sellers, equipment suppliers, food distribution centres, cuisine chat forums, etc. This widens your social circle. Every new skill gives you the head start to learn adjacent skills. For example, if you learn to do sound

---

[5] Airhart, Marc. 'Learning Expands the Brain's Capacity to Store Information', The University of Texas at Austin: College of Natural Sciences, 23 February 2018, https://tinyurl.com/z65kkpwz. Accessed on 4 April 2022.

recording, you would also learn to digitally manipulate sound, learn sound balancing, digital encryption, mixing music, etc. New skills are important to rejuvenate our fading interest in what we do currently. This is especially true during our Life 2.0. Boredom and fatigue are two illnesses nobody wants to court. A new skill opens up new pathways to engage us, just like the effect fresh air can have on us. There are some people who convert their learning into an ability to teach. If you self-taught something, you must be confident of guiding others too! Thus, we do not need external recognition or monetary rewards for learning new skills. At the stage of Life 2.0 or later, we must know how to pep ourselves up.

I know of people learning to drive or cook at 60—and that too proficiently! Some skills, especially related to languages, get harder to acquire as you grow older. It is not necessary to start learning a new skill during Life 2.0 or 3.0, but somehow when things are going smooth and are on cruise control, the urge to do so is muted. It seems to pick up vigour at the right time and moment. Life 2.0 is a great point in life to do this.

As Life 2.0 beckons, some of us are likely to seek new careers or professions. There are many reasons why we do this, not in the least due to a lack of satisfaction in what we have done so far. We may also resent our relative progress that leads to the idea that there are greener pastures elsewhere. New learning missions could be the prelude for some career changes—from corporate to academia, from working to studying further, from a corporate career to one in fine arts, etc. The interest that these new skills generate in us may impact our professional goals as well. A friend of mine was a successful corporate executive for over 20 years. As a new interest, he started to coach students on market research techniques and practical wisdom. He got his feet so wet in the process that he decided to leave his job and enrol for a PhD to transition to a university teaching role in his fifties! Learning new skills is also an experience by itself. Millennials tend to choose experiences over assets (holidays instead of motorcycles). Living to experience is, thus, its own compelling thought. Many of us, in our fifties or sixties, have always prioritized tangible financial and physical progress at the cost of new and memorable experiences. The pursuit of a new skill will bring us into contact with a new ecosystem, people, rules, routines, discoveries and perhaps even mindsets. Such a journey is precious for our transformation. The Canadian musician Leonard Cohen's first profession was as a novelist and a writer.[6] It was not till he turned 50 that his music career took off and his ultimate legacy of being a famous musician was cemented. He did dabble in music when he was 33, and it is believed that he worked on his musical prowess even while pursuing his writing. So, if you are a multi-dexterous person, as some people are, look after your second and third interests as well. They may become your primary vocation at some point in Life 2.0.

---

[6]Leonard Cohen, https://tinyurl.com/2t5kpkfu. Accessed on 4 April 2022.

It may not be all rosy when we move out of our comfort zones. A new skill will test us more than academic subjects did when we were young. Our brain gets conditioned to a certain way of learning, over time. A new skill may require a new way to analyse, interpret and apply it. For example, if you seek to study a new language, you may intuitively think of watching videos and try reproducing the contents. The better recommended method may be to first understand the structure of the language, its differences from the languages we know, some essential elements of grammar and maybe some training of the voice production apparatus. All this would need classroom learning, but we may be unprepared for it in Life 2.0. Tucking our tails between our legs and reimagining ourselves as students is the hardest thing to do. This will determine how we can pick up new skills systematically. I have recently published a book on habits for smart skill-building that reflects on the skill-learning capacity and rules.[7]

It is advisable to zoom in on one or two new skills at a time so that the learning is more focused and the practice, more distributed rather than crammed. Equally, we must measure our own progress against the lessons and stop at the right time if our progress shows adverse trends when compared to our efforts. In doing so, it is better to seek a benchmark of people at par with our calibre. Motivation experts will tell you that favourable interim results of any

---

[7]Shankar, Bala. *The Twelve Habits of Smart Skill-Building: A Code for the Reskilling of You*, Penguin Random House SEA, 27 September 2021.

new effort often spur you to continue the learning process. This is also the fundamental theory in rehabilitation from health issues. The rate of progress is not linear and may happen in spurts.

Do hobbies count as a new learning? Yes, provided they lead to a new skill. Many 'green-fingered' experts sprout at a later age, when they start mending a small private garden initially and develop the interest to grow it further, including acquiring knowledge on soil, plant growth science, nutrition and plant care. Similarly, writing a blog or a company newsletter could lead to a more active writing path as the interest grows. The key is to sustain and build the skill to a significant, measurable and noticeable level. We must be honest in the assessment of our skills. For instance, Min Bahadur Sherchan, a Nepali mountain climber, became the oldest person to climb the Mount Everest at the age of 77 in 2008 (although his record has been broken since then). Until he achieved this feat, his climbing hobby had been limited to accompanying climbers as a Sherpa. He sought to reclaim the record eight years later, only to perish at the ripe old age of 85 at the Everest base camp. Thus, Min brought together his general interest, occupation (as a Sherpa) and instinct to turn his life-long hobby into a new skill journey. No age is too late to give finality to a skill that you keep building.

How many new skills can we learn in Life 2.0 or 3.0? The simple answer is: as many as you desire and can devote time to. A range of 3–8 significant new skills is very much possible in a span of about 10–20 years. The key, therefore, is to start early—as soon as you reckon you are ready for Life 2.0.

How to get started?

There is a process you may wish to follow to get started (it is not rocket science). Identify the five things you are very good at and five things where you would rank very low (as compared to your contemporaries). Map each to a skill. Five is just a convenient number—it can be more or less. Which one of the five poor skill areas would you like to improve and how can your five strengths help in that journey? Some people go back and choose a skill that they always wanted to learn or gave up on early.

Here are some other questions to think about when deciding to start acquiring a new skill:

- What is the best way to learn the new skill (self-teaching, paid tutor, unpaid friend, enrolment to a formal course, online lesson)?
- How much time do you think you need to allocate per week or month to acquire this skill (corroborate this with others who may also be acquiring the skill)?
- And, finally, how much time are you willing to put aside per week or in a month for this skill?

If you have prepared this much and feel motivated, start with baby steps but keep the first milestone in view. This milestone can be the level of progress you wish to reach in

60 or 90 days, for example. Such milestones are important for conforming to a disciplined schedule of learning and practice. Another way to keep up your commitment to the new pursuit is by talking about it with like-minded friends and sharing learning styles, challenges, milestones, tips, etc. At some point in time, force yourself to do a demo in front of another person—spouse, a friend, a group. This is a good surrogate for a public performance and helps you work towards the event, like toddlers performing a concert! If there is an option to acquire a formal certificate in the skill, consider applying for it since it can further push you towards perfecting it. At all points, be realistic and honest with yourself and your efforts. Remember that you may need to put in more effort than a much younger person. Sticking to a routine helps with this. One reason to take up more than one activity is that if circumstances force you to give up one, you are not shattered. While a 'black belt' may not be everyone's dream, it is better to aim for a mid- to high-level of skill in whatever you choose. Once you feel you have reached an 'acceptable' level, find a way to put it into your activity cycle lest you lose the skill for lack of practice.

Impacting Society

No work is insignificant. All labour that uplifts humanity has dignity and importance and should be undertaken with painstaking excellence.

—Martin Luther King Jr.

THE MANDATES: COORDINATES OF A NEW JOURNEY 23

I wish to start this section with a real story. One of my classmates shaped his academic pursuits for the business world, with an engineering degree and a premier MBA. He ran his own engineering enterprise successfully for many years. When his son returned after his education in the US, he took over the father's business. In his late fifties, my classmate made an astounding switch to practising law, which he had trained for earlier in his life. However, he decided to focus his energies on Public Interest Litigations (PILs), fighting for social causes in the difficult legal environment of India. This is an unpaid job! In 2016, he secured a landmark judgement where the court directed the government to monitor waterbodies to prevent encroachment that eventually depletes their storage capacity and leads to water scarcity.[8] If you have noticed, this activity has no financial gain and there is a full-time involvement in this occupation. Where do we stand vis-à-vis involvement in activities that may not benefit us directly? And to what extent do we want to be involved with them?

Bill Gates is among the most successful entrepreneurs, creating one of the world's top companies (Microsoft), which led to his net worth climbing to briefly touch USD 100 billion by the age of 45.[9] In 2000, he decided to float

---

[8] M, Akshatha. 'Meet the Chennai crusader who has filed 20 PILs in two years!', *Citizen Matters Chennai*, 28 July 2017, https://tinyurl.com/5e3ax25w. Accessed on 4 April 2022.

[9] Vega, Nicolas. 'The world's 10 richest people added $402 billion to their fortunes in 2021. Here's whose net worth grew the most', *CNBC Make It*, 30 December 2021, https://tinyurl.com/35zm84vs. Accessed on 4 April 2022.

the Bill & Melinda Gates Foundation that went on to become one of the largest privately funded foundations (with estimated assets of USD 50 billion).[10] The foundation, as everyone knows, works to improve education and healthcare in under-developed societies. In this anecdote, Gates' age when he made this change—45—comes to the fore! We have already talked about Mahatma Gandhi and Abraham Lincoln's age while analysing their transitions. Similarly, why did Bill Gates decide to transition to full-time philanthropy at the age of 45?

Impacting society is probably everyone's wish and saves me the job of convincing anyone of its legacy potential. It may not need a sales pitch, but it does need a discussion. For instance, have you articulated the need to be useful to society? Did you reflect on the vast disparity in the lives that we lead and the lives of many other underprivileged people? Have you generated any ideas to help us do our bit to address this situation? What have you done with those ideas? More importantly, how far did you go? Bill Gates evangelizes his current interest through his foundation's activities wherever he goes much more than his professional passion of computing or the company he created. His engagement is, thus, manifold—through finances, management and mobilization of opinion and persuasion for change.

We may not realize how much we can impact people with our words and deeds (and by corollary, how much we

---

[10]'Foundation Fact Sheet', Bill & Melinda Gates Foundation, https://tinyurl.com/mrywx49c. Accessed on 4 April 2022.

do not). Humanity, unfortunately, does not create everyone as equal nor does everyone receive the same opportunities. Unequal abilities plus varying circumstances make for uneven outcomes. Over time, such inequality only grows. We have all witnessed such inequality, and we let it pass by us every day. Should we choose to be mute spectators or could we do something, however small that effort may be?

The circles of interest

Who do we impact in our lifetime? In a simplistic sense, all of us have three circles (not necessarily equal sized) of interest, with some overlaps.

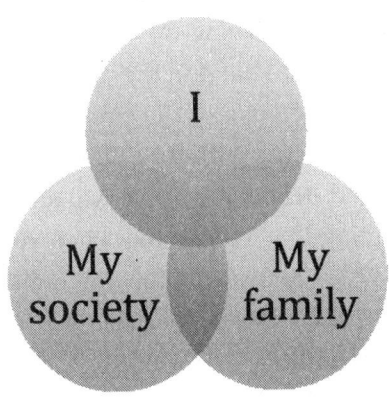

The first is 'I', the second is 'my family' and the third is 'my society'. The family could include extended family in some cases. Everything that we do has the inherent motive of serving one or more of the circles. We seek a stable financial situation so that we can have all the comforts, and so can our family. Similarly, we work to maintain a clean and hygienic environment around our homes for our own health and well-being, besides being considerate to our neighbours and the society at large. We drive carefully to protect our lives, the lives of our co-passengers and the rest of the road traffic. Most pursuits, thus, have multiple beneficiaries. Unsurprisingly, there is a sequence of interest as well—I, my family and my society, in that order. There may be minor exceptions to this universal rule. The more striking thing to note is that this sequence changes over time and along with it, the sizes of our circles change. One clear example is the change in our interest in children from when they are born to when they go to school or the later stages of them growing up to be adults. There is no precise mathematical split for the three circles, but they are never equal—even two of the circles may not be equal, and they grow or shrink with time. These changes are both subconscious and deliberate, as we will see later.

The first thing that strikes you when you are ready to embrace a new life is that in your single-minded focus on the self and perhaps the family, your societal obligations are reduced to nothing or serviced at a minimum. This is, of course, not true for a small number of people who dedicate their lives to social causes from very early days. Social work is somehow given lower priority, but it continues to be a buried need or desire. Our social utility in Life 1.0 is often restricted to some monetary donations—maybe to the Salvation Army—the odd visit to an orphanage, etc. It is not seen as an activity that can impact our life outcomes. When the expectations change, the motives change too.

The world needs us

The world around us is looking for people to play larger roles—financially, physically, managerially, emotionally and entrepreneurially. We are constantly being made aware of acute poverty, hunger, lack of shelter, sanitation or drinking water, infant mortality, illiteracy, etc. Besides these major social issues, there are several smaller and local social needs that are neglected for a number of reasons. Most people's hearts would melt upon witnessing these scenes, and at least mentally, they would want to help. However, only some actually do.

Hierarchically, most people are willing to donate money (some less and others more generously) at the very least. The next possible add-on to our societal engagement is a few hours of volunteering during our spare time. At the next level, people may lend their time to contribute as a manager of some sort, bringing their expertise to running not-for-profit organizations, serving on committees or delivering and organizing talks. The very nature of the volunteering and managerial intervention makes the commitment fluid and, therefore, has sustainability and scale questions.

For instance, you may spend two to three hours every weekend willingly teaching mathematics to young children.

Can you do it for all 52 weeks (without holidays or personal days off)? Can you scale it up to eight hours if the situation demands it or if more children come forward to receive such help? We justify our relatively limited engagement as the best possible way for us to contribute, keeping our skills and time in mind. Most people stop at this level, as they may not be willing to cut out some other activities to increase this engagement further. Some may see this as an excuse. Juggling our engagement in all the three circles is, of course, a challenge, mentally and in terms of time. We often punch well below our weight when it comes to engaging in activities that impact society. But the world is poorer because of that, and so are we.

A few people lend their energy in an entrepreneurial way, helping other people start a social enterprise or finding significant funds to run it. It is clearly a sustained commitment of a higher order. We tend to go through these phases, as perhaps some form of guilt of not playing our role in the society and being selfishly anchored to our personal and family needs catches up with us.

Aligning with the new activity

How do we change the level of engagement in activities that impact society? We need to raise our contributions noticeably and sustainably. While choosing an activity or a cause, it is perfectly fine to dovetail the choice to our context (time, money, location, skills, passion, etc.). This will be an easy start that we can sustain. A senior from my business school devotes several hours a week to a Bengaluru-based voluntary organization that rescues kids who run away or get separated from their homes, provides them temporary shelter, food and counselling, and eventually traces the parents to arrange a reunion.[11] This organization has rescued over 77,000 children across 11 Indian states, mainly from railway stations. They operate temporary stay centres, often in small government buildings, initiate the search for their parents, by and large, with the help of the local police and then reunite the children with their parents. The organization also tracks the reunited children post the reunion and ensures legal protection under child protection laws. My senior, with his business management degree and exposure, acts as the wise counsel in the organization. He helps plan new and effective strategies, and establishes best practices that contribute to a better result for the runaway kids. Thus, he brings his knowledge, time, location proximity and managerial and people skills to the table. It is a low-cost model, therefore, it does not demand a high financial commitment, and yet, it has achieved significant outcomes for the society.

It is never too late for you to start impacting society in a sustained and serious way. There are two types of serious involvement. First, you dedicate all (or most of) your energy to a cause or an organization that is working towards some human support or improvement outcomes.

---

[11]Society for Assistance to Children in Difficult Situations, https://tinyurl.com/yckwat6b. Accessed on 4 April 2022.

Second, your commercial entity (job, enterprise) has a social angle to it and you are actively directing your enterprise's social agenda. In my own circle of acquaintances, there are a variety of examples of serious involvement in a social cause. A friend of mine works in an influential position at a bank, and he guided his employer to a significant sponsorship of Paralympic athletes. He has shown a constant passion to get such efforts to higher levels.

A former colleague, after retiring early from a successful corporate career, is now working full-time, pro bono, as a senior director at a large foundation that brings real laboratories to students in government schools in remote villages via the mobile laboratory model.[12] The foundation has 210 mobile laboratories (some on bikes too) and reaches out to over 10 million children across 19 states in India. My former colleague is clear that he does not want to be paid for his time and does this as a full-time job. This is a rather serious commitment, given the size and scope of the operations of the foundation. He obviously lends his managerial and private-sector expertise as well so that the organization is more efficient and impactful.

These are significant examples of mid- to high-levels of engagement in matters that affect our society. They also offer a spectrum of how and where we can offer our help. You may not have thought of many of these aspects, but at some point, we grow apprehensive that our remaining lives

---

[12] Agastya International Foundation, https://tinyurl.com/mryct7as. Accessed on 4 April 2022.

may not be enough to carry out these activities satisfactorily. We also tend to mull over such decisions for years rather than trying to take baby steps towards them. Talking about making an impact on society or processing the idea in our minds does not amount to actually doing something. I have, unfortunately, come across several people who are stuck in this transit lounge for a long time.

There may be a few genuine reasons for such hesitation. The work culture of some social support organizations leave a lot to be desired, which can discourage people from supporting them. However, despite news about misappropriation, hidden agendas, scepticism, poor funding or managerial strength, many non-government organizations (NGOs) across the world carry out amazing transformational work. The fact that many of these NGOs are small-scale is another difficulty in ensuring benefits for larger sections of the society. Many projects have gone on for decades with some impact but without large-scale eradication of social ills or sustained changes. Thus, there is an important, unmet demand for a holistic approach to NGO interventions, with leadership inputs and institutional mechanisms. Many of us who have had such exposure in the private sector have the ability to steer such a mission. How many of us will do it? It depends on how we redraw our circles. It also depends on how much we want to take control of our conscious efforts in this direction.

My interest in such activities was piqued at some point when I chanced upon some different opportunities. I consider the school that I co-founded in 2008 as partly a social-impact enterprise, even though there is a business aspect to it. Our school offers high-quality private education at affordable fees. Our methods are all above board, including admission criteria (no management intervention or quota) and financial management. In the Indian context and even overseas, private school operations are not always clean and ethical. For over eight years, I have spent 20–30 pro-bono hours per week at the school, contributing in areas like long-term strategy, marketing, external liaising, etc. As graduates from the school leave with top achievements in academic and holistic aspects every year, you can imagine my sense of satisfaction. I am also associated with an organization in India for another activity. Under an ongoing programme, our private trust has provided scholarships to over 600 female students from rural areas in the vulnerable age group of 12–18, when they are most likely to drop out of school for a variety of reasons. This programme is now set to expand because we realized that we were able to make an impact and motivate the girls to insist on being educated till they finished high school, at the very least. Credit should be given to our partner organization at the ground level and their ability to identify and develop targeted programmes like these. There are further exciting extensions to this coming up. My wife and I go to the villages every year to meet and talk to the beneficiaries under the scholarship programme.

For a short period of about 18 months, I gave English lessons to a family of three children in an underprivileged society in Singapore. The parents of the children are uneducated and were unable to coach or monitor the children's progress. Along with my siblings, we instituted an endowment at our high school, which pays out some prizes to high-achieving students as well as a lump sum amount to a former teacher of the school. Most teachers tended to belong to the lower middle class in our days, and we know that they would have continued to be in financial distress with added health issues in their later days. We consider these as very small returns of the favours the school and the teachers did to us while we were in school. These are easy commitments that most people can take on, which could be seen as a basic effort.

What are the lessons that one learns?

The lessons that one can learn (I learned some too) through such social endeavours are:

- We need to start somewhere instead of intellectualizing too much. This is the bane of the inability to start something.
- We need to identify our niche and area of comfort that would also make a social impact.
- Unless you are an expert multitasker, it may be prudent to take up one or two aspects on which you can focus best.
- It may be a good idea to go beyond just writing cheques—only then is the commitment more

serious and satisfying. The experience of direct physical involvement is very different.

- Do something at a personal level, not just through your organization.
- Whenever possible, spare chunks of time to help organizations or causes. We tend to be frugal with sparing our time.
- Unlike a corporate setup, you may not need a long-term vision to get started. A small lane will lead you to bigger roads, if your mind is open.
- Keep a routine for social-support activities. This helps you make time and takes away any excuses for avoiding such activities.
- Do some basic research to identify the right causes where you can make the maximum impact.
- When choosing partners to work with, make sure you understand the motivations of the individuals and their organizations.
- For the reluctant starters, joining a buddy or another family member is a good solution.
- Don't compare your contribution to that of others, as each person's capacity, circumstances and goals are different.
- Be prepared for some disappointments, as outcomes are less important than the efforts or the purpose. Also, you may not be able to control all the variables in a social programme.
- Don't stop social engagement even under testing

circumstances. It is very easy to disengage when some other aspect of your life is under stress or when time seems to be short.
- Avoid publicity because it somehow takes away the satisfaction by highlighting a personal gain rather than a public good. Remind yourself that this is not about what you get from society but the other way round. Your pictures and media attention matter less than the ways in which you improve the lives of many unfortunate people. There is an Indian saying that is apt for this situation: the left hand should not know what the right hand gives!
- Motivate others around you to take up an appropriate social cause.
- Focus on your philanthropic pursuits as much as you do on your career or other interests.
- Walk away graciously after doing any such work.
- Reflect proudly on your contributions but never seek credit.
- Talk about your social activities with children at home to sensitize them early. Take them along on your support trips.
- Whenever possible, start training others so that you can ensure continuity.
- Document your work for posterity and for others to carry on what you started.

If you are a believer, this is the perfect method to build your karma. The rule of karma says that events and outcomes in your next life or rebirth are a function of the 'good deeds account' that you have maintained in your previous births. It is meant to act like a bank account transferred to the new birth. The Hindu and Buddhist religions are founded on this principle. Christianity also extols the virtue of compassion and helping others.

Like all activities in life, there is a time to reflect, seek feedback and decide on how we could impact society in the future. Further along this journey, we must evaluate our efforts, outcomes and feelings. This is necessary to either redirect the efforts or to scale them up, depending on your experiences. Share your experiences with others who have reached out similarly, as this can enrich both parties.

As our personal needs (and familial needs too) start reducing, the societal circle has the potential to fill the vacuum. To some extent, this is the key to thinking further about impacting society (see the section on decoupling finances and life, page 64). The problem, however, is taking the first step. An early start, even on a smaller scale, can lead to a more meaningful engagement at a later stage, directly benefitting from the trials and tribulations. The lever to make this change is squarely in our hands. So, just begin! Keep a scrapbook of your experiences for you to reflect on and share.

It is a no-brainer that the mandate for impacting society contributes directly to our legacies. Many philanthropists are more famous for their positive impact on society than their private or corporate achievements. John D. Rockefeller and

THE MANDATES: COORDINATES OF A NEW JOURNEY 37

the Rockefeller Foundation are classic examples. Not many may know that Rockefeller was also the most successful oil businessman of his time.

The youth are in it too...

I am perhaps a tad mistaken when I recommend this mandate for Life 2.0. Muhammad Yunus, Nobel laureate and famous Bangladeshi social reformer and inventor of the rural banking concept,[13] says, 'I'm encouraging young people to become social business entrepreneurs and contribute to the world, rather than just making money. Making money is no fun. Contributing to and changing the world is a lot more fun.'[14] If you wish to adopt this philosophy, you can impact society at any age. In the International Baccalaureate (IB) programme[15] that is gaining popularity among many parents and schools (our school offers this curriculum too), there is an in-built 'service' segment that students of grades 11 and 12 engage in for a certain period of time. This can be a good baptism into taking on greater tasks to better our society. There is also a lot more hope for higher participation from millennials and Gen Z as they seem to be more keenly interested in following their heart, including serving the

---

[13]Bank for the Poor: Grameen Bank, https://tinyurl.com/2p8m437s. Accessed on 4 April 2022.
[14]'Quote 133: Professor Muhammad Yunus, Young, Quotes', Yunus Centre, https://tinyurl.com/4zw4x7bw. Accessed on 5 April 2022.
[15]International Baccalaureate, https://tinyurl.com/bddkp9zn. Accessed on 4 April 2022.

society. For instance, Teach for America, is a two-year commitment that young graduates undertake for a nominal pay after their graduation to help improve educational equity and excellence in government and rural schools, largely serving low-income families.[16] The movement has had over 50,000 corps so far, and the benefits have reached over five million schoolgoers.[17] Such youth organizations for teaching exist in several other countries as well.

Revisiting Missed Opportunities

Use what talents you possess, for the woods would be very quiet if no birds sang there except those that sang best.

—Henry Van Dyke

Julia Child was a homemaker and enjoyed cooking at home for her foodie husband, Paul Child. This was until she decided, one fine day, to put some more meat into developing her skill for a larger pursuit. At the age of 49, she published her famous book on French cuisine, and from then on, she became the icon for French cooking in the US,[18] all achieved after she crossed 50. Child (1912–2004)

---

[16] Teach for America, https://tinyurl.com/mufeuy22. Accessed on 4 April 2022.

[17] 'Our Impact', Teach for America, https://tinyurl.com/3n5h9rrd. Accessed on 4 April 2022.

[18] 'Julia Child', *Encyclopaedia Britannica*, https://tinyurl.com/5n7zt2ja. Accessed on 4 April 2022.

won a Peabody, an Emmy and several other awards and recognitions, including having a rose named after her in the UK and an exhibit at the National Museum of American History. How did Child's latent interest in cooking turn into a strong desire to go out and seek a path-breaking opportunity? Had the opportunity been staring her in the face all along?

We are human and, hence, can't do justice to all opportunities that we get in life, even among the ones that we recognize. Time, priority, low willingness or sheer laziness put many opportunities away from our radar quickly. Some opportunities are missed without recognizing, others are let off without due consideration and many others are allowed to slip away because we believe that we have other priorities. Some, however, come back, giving us a second chance. When we reach the crossroads of an impending Life 2.0, it may be a perfect moment to reflect on the path so far—the accomplishments, the failures, the lessons learnt, the impact they had on our intellect and behaviour, etc. Most interviews of famous achievers have a stock question: 'If you were to do it again, what would you change?' The reality of life is that you never encounter the same situation twice in your life. Even if the situation is similar, you are not the same person, and the environment around you that can impact the outcome would have changed.

It is still a useful, if hypothetical, exercise to revisit some key inflection points in your life and assess the outcomes. Introspection can lead to a new discovery that can influence the outcomes of our Life 2.0. They also often have a huge impact on how we make decisions and act in the future. In fact, such actions may also lead to a stunningly different legacy, as many late bloomers would affirm.

The questions that spotlight past opportunities

In our Life 1.0, we certainly focus on a few goals, sometimes almost exclusively. Does this lead to under- or no achievement in some of the other goals that we are expected to achieve or we would have liked to engage in? What are those areas of underachievement? Education, career, family, finances are some obvious items on the checklist. But we can go beyond them and explore some subtle emotive aspects as well. Here are some of the questions we may ask to assess Life 1.0:

- How well have we bonded with our spouse and children? It's never too late to address this question.
- How has our relationship with our parents changed over time? How do our parents see it?
- What is our identity (as opposed to status) in the immediate society that we belong to (work, friends, neighbours, professional circles, etc.)?
- What is our friendship quotient (not to be confused with Facebook friendships or followers), and how has it evolved?
- How do our children respond to us now? How have we impacted their childhood and adolescent years?

THE MANDATES: COORDINATES OF A NEW JOURNEY

- What are some of the virtues that we have embodied and some that we have failed to model enough?
- What are some opportunities that we would classify as ones that we missed terribly?
- What could be other goals that we would have set for ourselves in hindsight?
- What do we see in others that we perhaps did not explore for ourselves enough?
- What are the soft aspects of our character that remained unexplored?

These questions can also be worded as: What did we fall short on or miss in Life 1.0? The responses to this question can be classified into two levels: mild and strong.

Take a sheet of paper and write all the missed goals, underachieved missions, unattempted pursuits and intriguing quests in your life that you have encountered. Casual hobbies like solving crossword puzzles are not intended to be included in this discussion, but if you are thinking about challenging the Guinness Record for crossword solving speed, surely yes! Rate your performance on each of these on a scale of 1 to 5 (with 5 being the best). What does your scorecard look like? What are the areas where you scored around 3? From these, are there some where you would have liked to achieve a 4 or a 5?

Billionaire Bill Gates opened up about his biggest personal regret being that he didn't learn more about global inequality until later in life. He feels that being aware of the problems humanity faces in the early years makes one better equipped to work towards solving them with more time on one's hands.

In 2011, former President Barack Obama helped (with US military assistance, of course) remove the Libyan dictator Muammar Gaddafi from power. While he knew intervening was the right decision, he regrets his lack of a follow-up plan for the scenario after the event. Libya was thrown into turmoil after Gaddafi's removal, and the country is still recovering today. Obama said in an interview that his failure to plan for the day after the intervention was his worst mistake as president.[19] Did he have the opportunity to revisit it? You could say he always had it.

Missed opportunities can also take the form of missed learning (lessons), ignoring relationships, failing to balance various aspects of life, not grabbing at the chance to change lives (one's own or others') or passively maintaining the status quo when changes abound in our lives. Fortunately, these may not create serious consequences. Otherwise, we would be forced to respond. But that low threat of adverse consequences is also a disincentive.

In my own case, there are several aspects of relationships—with family and friends—that I could have perhaps been more attentive to. Maintaining friendships from college, supporting parents, being more involved with my daughter's school life, learning new languages, shedding some of my ultra-competitiveness at work, embracing

---

[19]'President Obama: Libya aftermath 'worst mistake' of presidency', *BBC News*, https://tinyurl.com/3whrk3a5. Accessed on 4 April 2022.

philanthropy earlier (who will disagree with Bill Gates' observation mentioned above?), travelling around the world earlier (gaining global exposure and widening my cultural sensitivities) are some areas where I would certainly rate myself 3 or lower. The learnings are obvious. Some are missed opportunities and a few do present themselves again in Life 2.0. Such reflections help us retool ourselves to achieve better outcomes, should we get another chance.

A distinction must be drawn between new experiences that you may seek and going back to old, missed opportunities. In the former, you probably never encountered something like it, or the pursuit never existed (space tourism, for example). We always seek and even enjoy new experiences as the river of life exposes us to such journeys, but we seldom look back at what we missed or did not attempt. Some may even think of this as a futile exercise. I don't think so. If we are willing to reflect, we could resurrect some of the missed opportunities. A good friend of mine adopted a child in his late fifties, as the couple did not have a biological child. The opportunity must have been knocking at his door for a long time, but not closing the door helped the couple. They are popular parents at their child's school for their progressive act. Other people adopt pets, something that they always wanted to. Such acts also reflect one's character and lead to new energies in Life 2.0.

> So many men and women in middle age share that they regret what they've missed out in life, by working so hard. They missed being in the fabric of their

children's lives. Or they missed the chance to have children. They missed the opportunity to build true intimacy and closeness with their spouses, family and friends. They missed experiencing adventure, travel, enjoyment, vitality, learning, spiritual growth—not having the chance to stop and relish life, nature, good health, peace, or relaxation. They missed so much and sacrificed so much to pursue work goals alone.[20]

We need to remember that we are the only stakeholder in this introspection. A second attempt at the pursuits that we underachieved in the first attempt is perhaps of consequence only to us. In some cases, these areas are so subtle, like our relationship with our parents that only we know how well or poorly we did and how we can visibly improve them. We are the only ones who are capable of reflecting truly and identifying reasons for our underachievement. In other words, if we have no interest in doing this, no one else will be interested either. This is not quite the bucket list that people often talk about. These pursuits give us more self-esteem and satisfaction than, say, visiting a wonder of the world or something similar. They may also be inherently difficult. Otherwise, we would have attempted them earlier.

Unless the pursuits become irrelevant over time, they always stay with us and, sometimes, remind us too. I have come across three categories of people in this context:

---

[20] Caprino, Kathy. 'The Top 5 Regrets of Mid-Career Professionals', *Forbes*, 16 October 2016, https://tinyurl.com/w2syd43r. Accessed on 4 April 2022.

- The eternal optimists: They do not give up on an idea but merely put it aside. They will go after it at some point. They have a persevering streak.
- The forgetful people: They are not capable of recalling enough from the past. They have a happy-go-lucky streak.
- The apathetic people: They do remember missed opportunities but couldn't care less. There could be several reasons for such apathy. These people have a minimalistic or low-effort streak.

Who do you identify with by and large? We are our own slaves and masters, and revisiting a missed mission is very much in our hands. Our personality may provide the clue to our inclination.

My father-in-law completed his PhD in chemical engineering from the prestigious Indian Institute of Science in the 1960s and had a very bright career in academia, research and corporate technology. There wasn't a ton of money, but he accomplished a lot professionally. As he was retiring, his instincts turned him to financial investing, something he had attempted half-heartedly earlier and had not succeeded at. With more time in hand, he learnt the tricks of the investment trade (he was an exemplary lifelong learner). In a decade, he grew his portfolio five times, beginning with mutual funds and eventually doing intra-day online trading of equities. At his peak, he had at his fingertips the stock and earnings information of about a hundred companies and was ready for any discussion on the investment landscape and the merits of equity A vs equity B! He left his chemical engineering brain behind and threw himself into learning investment strategies and opportunities (the common thread being a logical and mathematical mind). The final decade of his life was almost fully and gainfully spent in this hobby-turned-expertise. In fact, it singularly kept him going in his last phase as he battled a terminal illness.

In another astonishing case of revisiting a missed goal, in 2015, three professors from Hamburg University's medical faculty travelled to Dr Ingeborg Syllm-Rapoport's private room in East Berlin to test her on the work she had done in pre-war Germany, and after conducting a satisfactory viva-voce, awarded Dr Ingeborg, a PhD at the age of 102![21]

This and other examples of revisitors—the octogenarian mountain climber, the 70-year-old first-time author or the retiree who learnt coding or programming are the people who have gone back to trying again. They embody the belief that a relevant goal is always within one's reach. Defeat is not a part of their dictionary. They can be role models for other less industrious people.

The essence of Chapter 8 of the Bhagavad Gita is: never give up on yourself. This means that we are always capable of achieving better things, if only we seek those higher achievements, learn from previous mistakes and wipe out our ignorance.

---

[21] Grieshaber, Kirsten. 'Denied under Nazis, 102-year-old Jewish woman gets doctorate', *Boston Globe*, 9 June 2015, https://tinyurl.com/3fu3zsts. Accessed on 4 April 2022.

I revisited a couple of things in Life 2.0 and reintroduced them in my agenda. I revived my old tryst with classical music. As a youngster, I had put in little effort into this activity, which resulted in my underachievement as a likely performer. I renewed my engagement with classical music a good 20 years later as an organizer and a once-in-a-while performer, combining religion, history and music. I am still in the early days of this new effort. As an extension of this activity, I leant into writing about music. I also recalibrated the way in which I used to network, thanks to all the electronic tools and platforms that are now available to us. By contrast, I wasn't too far from being a recluse in Life 1.0. The early results of revisiting networking in a new way have been encouraging, as I am visibly engaged with a much larger group of friends and acquaintances, and am trying to attach myself to groups with common interests (many in Life 2.0 may be doing this as well). What we share is worth a lot more than what we know. Getting past the banal social media 'sharing' instinct is, of course, a challenge.

The purpose of revisiting missed opportunities

Revisiting previous underachievements or ignored opportunities gives us a chance to:

- Restore the goals from Life 1.0, if doable in Life 2.0 and if we want to pursue them (read about reassessing goals in our next section, page 49).
- Go about them differently from Life 1.0, based on

the lessons learnt and new life experiences gathered.
- Improve the power of true introspection (a skill we will need badly in the middle and later stages of life).
- Avoid regrets (at the Life 2.0 crossroad, these could weigh us down).
- Revitalize our sense of purpose and achievement; add new doses of expectation and vitamins to our routines.
- Be a role model to our children and others around us for trying and not giving up. The German researcher who got her PhD at the age of 102 is one such person.
- Reassess our current capabilities vis-à-vis our previously judged levels (many improve naturally with age and maturity). Internet tools have levelled the playing field for many activities that we may want to pursue as adults or later in life.
- Discover the meaningfulness of some activities that once seemed banal or inconsequential (spiritual engagement is one example).
- Enjoy the fruits of something that we achieve with self-motivation and perhaps with self-directed efforts.
- Remind ourselves that we are never too old (some psychologists even suggest this as a mantra to slow down mental ageing). Sudoku addicts will endorse this.
- Evolve in life as new methods create new ways to achieve old missions (we will discuss this in the next section).

- Keep ourselves fit, mentally and physically (atrophy is the worst form of becoming or feeling redundant faster).

A good way to start revisiting missed opportunities is to draw up a cheat sheet of significant things that you think you have underachieved. Don't be surprised if the list is long—it is a good reality check. Applying a criterion based on what is still meaningful to you and what looks doable (you may not be able to become a doctor in Life 2.0), choose one or two that you can rely on yourself to persist in—the outcomes may come slowly in some cases, especially if it involves the body. Celebrate all outcomes because that is an impetus to keep exploring further. It also tells people around you that you are the same lively, busy and persevering person that you had been in Life 1.0, even if that is not the main purpose of the pursuit. This indirectly impacts our legacy—you would certainly be rated and known as a valiant trier for life!

Reassessing Goals

Whatever you can do, or dream you can, begin it. Boldness has genius, magic, and power in it.

—Johann Wolfgang Von Goethe, German literary celebrity of the eighteenth century

Our lives seldom operate without goals. Some call it dreams, some say purpose, others may even equate it to wishes. The definitions are not important, but just the fact that we seek to do something (and not do some others) at all points of time in our lives. What originates that desire is also not that important. We need to recognize that there is never a journey without a destination in mind. Goals are synonymous with destinations. They may or may not be explicitly stated.

Dr Raghuram Rajan was an acclaimed economist and a tenured professor at the prestigious University of Chicago Booth School of Business for many years. He was also the chief economist at the International Monetary Fund for four years. As a successful economist and finance expert, he accumulated several laurels in the US, where he lived. He then switched his goals and joined the Indian government in 2012 (at the age of 49) and went on to become the governor of the Reserve Bank of India (a position similar to the head of a country's central bank) for three years. The two careers are worlds apart in every sense. Some media coverage reported that he was diving into the 'pressure cooker'. He also said that he was not looking to win many Facebook 'likes' at his new job.[22] What was his motive in making such an unlikely switch from a well-settled and famed career? What prompted him to reassess his goals?

---

[22]Press Trust of India. 'Raghuram Rajan says RBI governorship not meant to win Facebook "likes"', *The Indian Express*, 4 September 2013, https://tinyurl.com/yvvvumzs. Accessed on 4 April 2022.

Goal-setting principles and practice

Life goals are set and reset continuously, most by design, but chance cannot be ruled out either. It is useful to analyse the goal-setting behaviour. Goal-setting is a task and skill that we pick up perhaps in our early teens (completing homework, practising a song, sending invites to friends for a party, packing for a tour, etc.). At that age, these consist of simple things for the near future (a day, a week or a month). The habit, however, picks up momentum at every subsequent stage of life. The first set of serious goals concern education, extracurricular interests and maybe long-term friendships, courtship and companionship. It then moves slowly to career, finances, asset acquisition (a two-wheeler, car, home), marriage, children, lifestyle, etc. Depending on how much you love to-do lists, you are likely to make them in great detail, including target dates, etc. Others are likely to keep their goal-setting as a fuzzy file in their brain—fuzzy in terms of the goal and the timing. For example, we are capable of generating and storing goals like 'read about the importance of the Vedas' or 'sort out music collections'. Both have no specific milestone or timing. I know of some people who have a goal of 'starting to invest' and have not acted on it for over three or five years! The informality in personal goal-setting is perhaps a universal phenomenon and, therefore, has implications for Life 2.0.

At the risk of generalization, I would reckon that until a certain stage in life, money, career and family are everyone's dominant goals. There is a step-wise approach to these goals.

Once we reach a certain step, we reset to aim for the next step, and so on. For example, after you buy a home, you will probably reset to buy a bigger, better or a second home a few years down the line. Similarly, career goals start with initial objectives like getting a managerial position to get higher responsibilities, position and power. Family goals are likely to include the number of children, the nature and style of relationships to be maintained with one's immediate family (parents, etc.) and with a close circle of friends. There may be other social, recreational and financial goals (investments) as well.

Is this all a single track with no U-turns or side lanes? I have come across some very interesting goal resets. For instance, a friend started off as an accountant but started disliking it soon. Then, he switched to investment banking at a large global bank, which he enjoyed for a number of years before he got bored again. This time, he transitioned to university teaching, and to fortify his credentials, enrolled for a PhD programme in his forties! The required drive to act on these goals came automatically, and he is currently a professor who holds a PhD. He says this is the job he always thought he would enjoy! That's three or four turns within 20 years. The good thing for him was that he could identify his next goal, make the necessary switch and be dogged about achieving it. We often get confused between what we want to do and what we want to own or possess. That is a fundamental reason for why we keep misfiring our arrows.

If you notice the range of goals in the first few decades of life, they are essentially about getting more of everything—education, money, career, recognition, social status, etc. In the normal course of life, there is less qualitative difference (there is a quantitative difference, for sure) in many of the aspects. Thus, salaries rise from X to 5X or 10X, cars evolve from pre-owned hatchbacks to mid- or top-of-the-range ones, homes graduate from rented apartments to posh, large, owned apartments (with an upgraded locality), appliances and other comforts move in tandem, schools for children reflect one's better career status, and so on. The achievements may be somewhere on this spectrum for different people. Is there an ultimate logical destination? For example, if you are a vice president of a business or own a Toyota Corolla or Camry, is there some more distance for the goals to go? How and when do we begin to address this issue?

Some would say yes to both the questions posed above—maybe they want the CEO position and a BMW 7 series. One may need to do nothing more than stay in the carousel. However, at the point where Life 1.0 seems to be running out and a transition appears to be looming (even if it is not triggered by an event), do you want to reassess your goals—either in terms of magnitude or the very goals themselves? Is personal wealth of 2 million dollars more significant than 1.5 million dollars? Numerically, yes, but what if we are considering it from the point of view of redefining life? (More on this in the next section on decoupling finances and life, see page 64). What are meaningful revised goals? How are they different in character from the ones in Life 1.0? And how can they impact our lives? Mahatma Gandhi and Abraham Lincoln asked and addressed these questions seriously. The vast majority of us don't.

One is not just putting brakes on a range of old pursuits but perhaps engineering a subtle (or even pronounced) shift in the priorities and emphasis on different goals. Academics have a good system called 'sabbatical' that allows them to withdraw from their current work and professional routines, and use the time to redirect their efforts elsewhere—maybe teaching at another place that is totally different, embarking on some new research, travelling around the world, writing a book, setting up an institution or even helping a close relative in a start-up. How will we accept the idea of a sabbatical from our patterned life and goals? Would being a parent volunteer at the school of your child interest you more than a better paying job that allows you to travel? Would the prospect of knowing and engaging your child, and spending time with other children constitute a better way of spending the next six months of your life? Depending upon the culture and norms, children leave their parents between the ages of 15 to 20. After this, our family life is never full. The longer they stay away, the farther they move away from our lives. There is a short window of time when it is possible to develop a meaningful bond between parents and children while they are still at school. What is the best way to make sure that short span is not compromised by chasing goals that we have always chased?

How and when do new goals germinate?

While Life 1.0 is a journey of trying to achieve stated and unstated goals, our mindset towards the end of Life 1.0 undergoes an important transformation. For starters, the original goals and assumptions are up for debate. Depending on whether you consciously introspect or not, the mind starts questioning the old notions and canvassing opinions within for some new pursuits. The step-wise trend of goal-setting discussed earlier may never actually stop, but the transformation is inevitable. The previous goals take some turns and can become less conspicuous. Some people, however, are always on the pedal of goal-setting. Life 2.0 is a good point to review some or all goals. Here are some intentionally provocative questions to reflect upon at such a juncture:

- Do we want to continue to set hard goals as we did in our Life 1.0?
- What will be our new horizons?
- What areas will such horizons encompass?
- What will be their connection to our past or current goals?
- Will the new goals be congruent with or divergent from the previous ones?
- What implications does this shift have for our family and societal interface?

New goals are fantastic opportunities to diversify our personalities. Should we think of acquiring some new skills like learning a new language or playing the guitar, training for a marathon, doing a freelance activity based on our current expertise, etc.? It is assumed that many of the hard goals of career, money and family would have been somewhat realized (to different degrees of fulfilment, though) in Life 1.0, and the thrust of our goals subtly shifts in Life 2.0. It is a fact of life. We cannot survive just looking after a few areas all our lives. Even the Everest climber, however obsessed he or she may be with that goal, will wander to seek other interests and pursuits. A normal person's mind is a wandering one, seeking new engagements, challenges and discoveries. In some cases, such shifts have also resulted in second careers. Many in politics can vouch for this. Even Purandara Dasa sought a totally new goal and space that established his eventual legacy.

It is useful to understand the differences between our old goals and our potential new goals. Our old goals tend to be better defined (career position, income, etc.), have a certain roadmap and it is possible to estimate the efforts-to-results ratio. Newer goals like 'bonding better' or 'helping a sick friend' are not constituted by such finite elements—they lack a clear end point, we have a limited idea of the efforts required to achieve them, we have no assurance of being able to complete them and perhaps have to face more trials and errors ahead than well-chalked out plans. So, it is like diverting from a highway on to a gravel lane with no street signs. Yet, at the Life 2.0 point, the motivation to do some other things can hit you and, in fact, drag you further in that direction.

Another reason to reassess your goals in Life 2.0 is that some newly envisioned goals may need over 10 years to achieve—just ask entrepreneurs, musicians and artists who started working towards their goals later in life. Thus, it is necessary that you factor in the best years of your mental and physical health into the time schedules of such revised goals. You are not the same person at 60 as you are at 45, in every way!

In my situation, I was fortunate to have a couple of years of freedom from corporate life to spend quality time with my daughter before she went to college. I also reset some other goals, including financial ones, to discover the trade-offs that our corporate life normally forces us to accept. In hindsight, I am able to articulate that new experiences replaced money and quality replaced quantity in my goal-resetting. Inner satisfaction replaced externally recognizable feats and their symbols. Did it happen overnight? Absolutely not! The shift had been simmering within me for some time, but when some discontinuity happened (the point I call Life 2.0), it was easy to reset and embrace the new goals. The shake-up I encountered in 2006 was the God-given opportunity for me to reset goals and begin an almost new journey.

New goals

How do new goals germinate? It may be an organic or inorganic process. An example of organic connection is something that we have always wanted to do but could never prioritize, like becoming an expert in something! It could be to obtain a certificate in interior design—a subject that you are intuitively interested in. The inorganic path is more interesting. It could come from new knowledge, acquaintances or experiences. For example, you may have moved homes, and your new neighbour could be a fitness freak. He cycles 50 kilometers a week and perhaps runs a similar distance as well. He can, thus, convince or inspire you to get into a fitness regimen, as you now have a buddy to pursue this goal with. This may not have been a part of your goals before. However, it just happened to fall into your scheme of things. Many even take up fields like astrology or painting, based on having a minor interest in them and being exposed to a new environment.

The new goals can be congruent or divergent. For instance, you may move from a large corporate set-up to a start-up to experience its work culture—this would be a congruent or allied goal. If you leave the corporate world and take up farming or enrol for a full-time PhD programme, it is in the divergent zone. My experience is that the changes in goals are seeded in our minds much earlier than when we actually start pursuing them. Entrepreneurs think long before jumping into an initiative. People also debate their choices of goals with their close friends or family for some time before acting upon the changes. In this process, the evaluation of pros and cons, the what-if scenarios, the plan B in case of failure, etc., are regurgitated in our minds. The ultimate decision is often more gut-based than logical or based on spreadsheets. In some cases, the new goals exist alongside our existing goals but with some recalibration of time and effort. For instance, you may continue a day job but also start organizing a youth quiz on the weekends. Similarly, you may enrol to study astronomy at a local planetarium at night, twice a week. How we suddenly find the time and energy to engage in another substantive activity is not clear, but motivation neutralizes lethargy, diffidence and scepticism. We are drawn to the new goal by an inner sense or inspiration. It may also be a case of challenging ourselves to stay curious, fit or socially or mentally active.

In 2006, my business school batch celebrated its silver jubilee reunion. Nearly 120 of us, many with spouses, turned up, and many were meeting each other for the first time since leaving the institute. I managed to reconnect with many of my classmates who had changed careers, become entrepreneurs or academics, moved overseas, embraced life coaching, launched an NGO, initiated baby steps to becoming authors or were getting ready for the next undeclared move. Most of them were in their mid-forties. A significant number of my batchmates had shifted careers dramatically, even though many were still on a linear corporate track. The reunion gave me enough conviction that a dramatic reset of goals is more common than I had thought.

I must acknowledge that goal shifts in Life 2.0 are sometimes a function of reaching financial security or children growing up and being on their own or other such major life events. The greatest dampener to finding new goals is risk aversion. The risk of change in income, lifestyle, unlearning and new learning and other such disruptions can pull you back to your status quo. The idea of a settled life is both a blessing and a curse. Do you want to rock the boat of life or do you feel unchallenged and unmotivated with days and events repeating themselves ad nauseam? Everybody faces these dilemmas but very few act to change the status quo. The status-quoists are often the ones to lament later about the steps they did not take. Even risk experts fail when it comes to balancing personal risks. There are many stories of entrepreneurs who lost all their life savings before they became financially successful again. At the appropriate point, one force becomes greater than the other. Factors like your spouse's income, family circumstances, family backing, fall-back options or other risk mitigation strategies also govern the propensity to shift to new goals and accept their risks.

It is also possible that you move on to Life 2.0 goals, only to return to old goals after some time, either due to a lack of success in pursuing new goals or a lack of visibility on where the new goals will lead you. It may also be triggered by a sense of accomplishment in the new goal and a desire to return to the familiar. This is our 'safety first' gene in action.

Another friend who had several years of experience in the investment banking industry faced both these moments. A moment of new goal setting led him to start a fund management business of his own and a recoiling moment with his old goals led him to shut his new business down and return to his old career. Perhaps the results of his new goal had not been encouraging enough, even if the experience had been interesting. In today's diversified job market, such options to return to one's old goals are not difficult to find.

How to embrace new goals?

How do we initiate and manage goal changes rather than being mere spectators or being change-averse? To manage the transition to new goals, we need to answer the following questions:

- Do you have a good deal of clarity about what your new goal is (this includes specificity, purpose, timeframe, etc.)?
- Is the new goal a standalone goal, one that is interconnected with others or followed by subsequent goals? For example, you may start a weekend activity with the ultimate desire to step into it full-time.
- Are you pursuing this goal alongside an existing one? If yes, what is the balance of effort and priority that you seek?
- How different is the new goal from your current goals in terms of scope, effort, skills required or its end point?
- What implications does striving for this goal have on your life, money, location, family and other key aspects of your life?

- Are you doing this out of your own will or due to some external compulsions?
- What are the resources (time, money, education, etc.) you need to commit to have a reasonable chance of attaining the goal?
- How far and long are you willing to go down this new track? What is the timeline for it, if any? What is the stop-loss point at which you see yourself ending the pursuit of this goal?
- What do you plan to achieve or gain from the new goal(s)?
- What metrics would you use to judge whether the new goals have been achieved? How do you visualize the end point of this new goal?
- Do you want a fall-back option to help manage your risks?
- Have you thought through the new set of goals or have you set them based on intuition, impulse or a sudden urge?
- Are you doing this alone or do you have the benefit of role models and mentors?

Some may reckon that if we think so deeply (and critically), we will probably not make the move! That is fine, but the trouble is that when the moment for a shift in our goals passes, it adds to our list of regrets. A year from now, you shouldn't think that you should have started a certain activity last year, when the idea crossed your mind. Dealing with the moment squarely is, thus, a function of our risk-taking ability and clarity about the goal itself—why we are seeking it and what compromises are we willing to make as a consequence? I don't know about you, but I always evaluate new goal opportunities with a combination of intuitive desire and practical analysis, never just one of them. Doing it consciously is more beneficial than being swept up in the currents of a new idea. There is no perfect way to be prepared for changes in the new, fast-changing world order (both professionally and otherwise), but a sense of readiness is vital. This is also the premise of the eloquently written short book titled *Who Moved My Cheese?* by Dr Spencer Johnson, which has sold over 25 million copies.

When you shift your goals or are guided into shifting them (or chase additional concurrent goals), despite their disruptive nature, they bring opportunities to fulfil many of the other mandates in this book, such as impacting society, coaching and sharing, building social assets, decoupling finances and life, etc. These linked opportunities could lead to a new platform from where you can reshape your identity or legacy. That's what Dr Rajan would reckon he achieved through his switch to the top administrative role in the Indian economy. For many, new goals activate one's persona outside of their professional identity and sow the seeds for building a legacy. For instance, setting up the Bill & Melinda Gates Foundation is a new goal that allowed the billionaire to carve out a different legacy.

Decoupling Finances and Life

A childhood friend is a practising doctor. He has served in the government medical service for over 30 years. The salary in government service jobs is perhaps 50 per cent lower than private hospitals or personal practice. Yet, he chose this career option and stuck to it for almost the entire duration of his career. He has been living a very good life (apparently contented) with his doctor wife and a daughter, who completed her PhD in the US. My friend has had most of the comforts we all have. Perhaps he bought his first car a few years later than some of us. I am not sure what he lost by accepting a lower income, while all his contemporaries earned maybe two or three times more. You probably have seen many such examples in your lives. I am not suggesting that everyone should do this. Nor is this an attempt to promote a minimalistic lifestyle or living on shoestring budgets. Setting aside our default judgment of such people not being wise in terms of money, the more curious question to ask is: is it possible to decouple finances and lifestyle, happiness or satisfaction? It does seem so.

The life–money nexus

'Are we living to earn or earning money to live?' is a question that is answered differently depending on who you talk to. Many may not even be clear about its import. In modern life, money has taken centre stage. Our finances and standard of living are inseparably linked. In fact, our financial outcomes determine our ranking in the pecking order. But the curve is not linear all the way. At some point, the standard of living does not change even with more disposable income. This point is different for different people. It can also shift if our desired standard of living changes. If you are used to public transport but wish to migrate to private taxis, your income requirement goes up. Thus, there may be several step-wise changes in the standard of living that lead to higher sufficiency points. Do not ask whether your quest for more income and savings continues unabated even beyond this sufficiency point, since that answer may be a firm 'yes' for most people. The more nuanced question is how will the way you lead your life change beyond this sufficiency point? Remember, the highest sufficiency point still guarantees your revised standard of life. This is not about the old question of whether money buys happiness. We will pass that question for now. Instead, the question is: what is the finance–life balance you seek? Far from being a philosophical question, it's the most practical assessment of this delicate dilemma.

Let us imagine an individual with an income of USD 30,000 a year (please substitute equivalent amounts in your context). With this income, she and her family of four live in a rented home and pay for all their comforts and needs. Now, imagine her income increases to USD 60,000 per year. Her lifestyle upgrades to owning a house (she can now afford the mortgage payments), she indulges in a few simple luxuries, goes on an annual holiday, etc. Subsequently, her salary increases to USD 120,000 a year, and she makes similar upgrades, including buying a premium car, and so on. Now, what happens when she starts getting paid USD 240,000 a year? What are the things that will change and what won't? More crucially, where is the pause or end point in this? In arithmetic terms, how does the additional USD 210,000 from the beginning contribute to improving one's life (not just comforts but mental and physical well-being)? This scenario is not hypothetical, even if some adjustments are done for inflation.

The *Time* magazine reported in 2010 that '...no matter how much more than $75,000 people make, they don't report any greater degree of happiness,'[23] citing a study from Princeton University, conducted by Nobel laureates Angus Deaton (an economist who has extensively researched on positive psychology) and Daniel Kahneman (the author of the popular book, *Thinking, Fast and Slow*). The context of the study is the US but the idea applies everywhere. If you have been earning for 20 or more years, map the rise in your income and the increase in your life comforts. You may notice something unexpected—the break-up of the nexus between money and life, in figurative terms.

Writing for *The New York Times Magazine*, Charles Duhigg, a Harvard MBA graduate of 2001, shares his classmate's experience after 15 years of work: 'I feel like

---

[23]Luscombe, Belinda. 'Do we need $75,000 a year to be happy?', *Time*, 6 September 2010, https://tinyurl.com/yc8e6fhh. Accessed on 4 April 2022.

I'm wasting my life,' he told Charles. 'When I die, is anyone going to care that I earned an extra percentage point of return? My work feels totally meaningless.' While he was grateful for the incredible privilege of his pay (about USD 1.2 million per annum) and status, his anguish seemed genuine. 'If you spend 12 hours a day doing work you hate, at some point it doesn't matter what your paycheck says,' he told Duhigg. There's no magic salary at which a bad job becomes good. Duhigg's article was titled 'Wealthy, Successful and Miserable.'[24] This is a modern-day example of how your income and other needs are not necessarily linked over a period of time.

The money compromise

This is not a socialistic or anti-capitalist drumbeat and there is nothing wrong with seeking a continuously rising income or more money. It is the norm. But it may involve some of the following caveats (irrespective of whether you are fully cognizant of them):

- Accepting higher job responsibilities that may come at the cost of family or personal time
- Increased professional responsibilities that may increase stress levels and affect your overall health
- Disappointment and restlessness with the rate of

---

[24] Duhigg, Charles. 'Wealthy, Successful and Miserable', *The New York Times Magazine*, 21 February 2019, https://tinyurl.com/53zf3edh. Accessed on 4 April 2022.

increase in income (your desire vs the actual rise)
- Shifts in motivation and moods (parallel to the incomes)
- Acceptance of the higher risk that comes with higher rewards from investments, property deals, etc.
- Having to measure all trade-offs in terms of their impact on your income
- Lack of enthusiasm (or time) for other activities or pursuits
- Lack of diversity in your personality
- Obsession with a single financial goal (you become a slotting machine)
- Loss of sensitivity to the non-financial interests in life
- Feelings of being stuck in a quagmire with no chance of getting out—the more successful you are in making money, the deeper you dive into the rut
- Becoming greedy, often unconsciously
- Inviting behaviour that can potentially turn mildly or severely criminal (there are well-publicized cases of this and they happen alarmingly regularly)
- Potential erosion in your sensitivity towards people

I am not advocating for giving up on improving one's finances. From time to time, I have worked towards improving my finances too. But do you recognize these implications? How does your brain process such trade-offs, instinctively or otherwise? How do some people not get trapped by this chase?

You may be lucky to have landed in a career that has built-in increases in income, without any of the downsides mentioned above. However, I am sure that you are in a minority. For most people, such a situation is likely to last for certain periods, not forever. Some people are also fortunate to have sources of passive income, like investments or inheritances. We will focus on people whose time, life and money worked for and earned are substantially linked.

In the US and the UK, there has been a movement in recent years known as the Financially Independent, Retiring Early (FIRE) community. Laura and Brad Barrett from Virginia, USA, are a part of this community.[25] Brad says that the FIRE stage of your life can begin when your net worth is 25 times your monthly expenses (including all costs like mortgage payments, etc.). The exact number is arguable, but it is still an interesting concept. The couple clarified that they don't really want to stop working or earning but work and earn through opportunities that they want to pursue, perhaps for a lower salary and with more flexibility of time (with lower stress potential). This is a profound idea, but it needs to sink in! Similarly, over 25 years ago, my daughter's paediatrician, who trained to be a doctor in the US, would only work between 8.00 a.m. and 11.00 a.m. every day. His doors would be shut if you showed up at 11.05 a.m.! His consultation fees were on par with the standard rates. He was

---

[25] 'How This Couple Saved $1 Million in 11 Years and Became Financially Independent Before 40', Money, https://tinyurl.com/2dhxxksk. Accessed on 4 April 2022.

a very good professional and catered to a bunch of families regularly. His remaining time was spent on other interests, including being a pro-bono office-bearer of the local cricket association because he loved the sport. He was clearly an outlier and perhaps a precursor to the FIRE community!

The academic world is another perfect example. Salaries of teachers or university professors tend to rise slowly in the early years and perhaps peak at some point. Assuming that their salaries are generally beyond the sufficiency point, most academics tend not to focus on money. It is, at best, a subtext in their lives. Their professional goals and family objectives take over their lives. The academia has built-in breaks from their work in the form of sabbaticals, when they are free to do things other than their regular job, with some security on their basic income.

There are two challenges to managing the equation of life and money: capping your desired standard of living at some point (instead of continually moving the goal post) and graciously opting for a track that promises lower or no income raises (or even declines) in return for precious time to live life with a different set of pursuits. Life 2.0 presents the point at which this issue can be introspected and tackled.

Defining our relationship with money

'Nothing prepares you to see your bank account go down,' admits Khemaridh 'Khe' Hy, a Yale graduate and successful Wall Street banker, who turned into a freelancer at the age

THE MANDATES: COORDINATES OF A NEW JOURNEY 71

of 35![26] Hy is considered the Oprah of millennials due to his profound and bold outlook towards life and money. He has said that as long as he was a banker, he only saw the 'numbers', a euphemism for the financial goal that everyone like him chased. Scoreboards, status markers and the number of zeroes in the bank accounts became proxies for success until he chose to be jobless, in search of other things, including happiness. The story may be dramatic and out of the ordinary, but this dilemma hits most people at some point and leaves us with a conundrum.

When we try to reboot our attitude to finances, the relevant question to ask is 'What is our relationship with money?' There are several parts to this—from all-important and all-pervasive to least important and non-essential. The question is not whether finances are essential. They are, except for those who lead an ascetic life. But our relationship with money is determined by whether money comes first, last or somewhere in between on our list of priorities. As hardworking and competent people, many of us are convinced that we deserve to be compensated well financially. What happens if this is not the case for certain periods in our lives? Would you lose your mind over it? We must remember that *deserving and desiring money are two different things*. A sense of entitlement towards money is different from craving it. That is the essence of

---

[26] Long, Heather. 'Meet Khe Hy, the Oprah for Millennials', *CNN Business*, 31 December 2016, https://tinyurl.com/ytn8ve9h. Accessed on 4 April 2022.

the decoupling doctrine. If we understand this subtle but profound difference, we have moved beyond step one of this mandate. Our relationship with money is, and should be, defined by 'deserving money' but not 'lusting for money'. This is a fine line that is often crossed.

Many political and civil society leaders in the developed world have had two lives—one that preceded their political entry (as lawyers, businessmen, military officers, bureaucrats, etc.), and the political or public life that followed. Generally, people make more money in their pre-political lives than from their political careers. For instance, the US President draws a salary of about USD 500,000 a year, about half of what a young and successful Wall Street executive earns. Such political or public careers often mean more hours of work, less money, more challenges and less rest. Yet, people move from one life to the other, perhaps for the power, fame or some other attraction. It is clear to them that they need to divorce the money and the career goal (I am excluding the corrupt examples here). Every one of us may not be a political aspirant, but the point I am making is that legacy-making pursuits in Life 2.0 often come with a compromise on finances. It is, therefore, good to decouple them (and develop that mindset) earlier.

Recalling my situation in 2006, the loss of a steady salary after moving out of corporate employment did not trouble me enormously because the quest for the next professional pursuit dominated my mind. It was also comforting to know that we had already reached the sufficiency point (as defined by our own standards). Life suddenly stood on its own, not tethered to our income or job status. It happened quickly and did not give me us the time to ponder over it. It also mattered that neither my wife, Alamelu, nor I had, or have, a compulsive desire for more money. We have remained the same, before and after the shift. We aspired to live a middle/upper-middle-class life comfortably but with measured habits. It wasn't difficult to make the necessary adjustments, even though our family income swung from a certain amount to a quarter of that amount (although it eventually doubled). During this time, every expense was scrutinized before incurring it—this is my natural instinct anyway. That phase came and went! We could accept the change of scenario because we had started to prepare ourselves for decoupling money from life.

The story of another friend comes to mind. He had lost his job—a senior position in the IT industry. His family was small (the couple and a son) and I knew that their needs were reasonable and not extravagant. Due to the prevailing market conditions and his niche skills, he could not land a new job soon. We had some conversations at the time and I tried to counsel him with some other examples, including mine. His reaction was startling. He said he had not reached his wealth goals, even though he was comfortable except for some asset-related goals. He compared himself to another common friend who, despite freelancing, was estimated to have twice his net worth! I must admit I had not thought of that angle before. Do you get bogged down by such comparisons? It is vital to realize that comparisons are fraught with danger. My income and wealth will always be less than that of some people on the planet, maybe even lower than some people in my immediate circle of friends or people who have had similar education or career backgrounds. That's how the world is organized. Should it bother me? Should it, therefore, take my life away and put me back in the chase for money? How can I develop the equanimity required to accept my unique financial destiny? The answer to this lies in looking inward rather than out. Our reference point is inside us.

Defining the life vs finance landscape

This is a basic diagrammatic expression of the money vs life question.

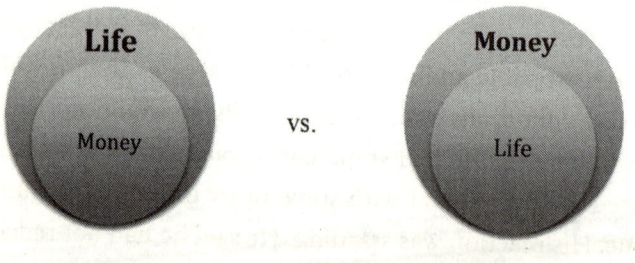

A simple model-building exercise can lead us to some guided thoughts:

- What is the standard of living you desire at your peak earning capacity?

- How does it translate to goods, services, experiences, activities, pursuits?
- What are the finances you think you need at a minimum for your sunset years?
- Why is substantially more income (above such needs) important to you?
- What is your emotional link to higher and rising incomes?
- What are the life possessions or experiences you are willing to sacrifice if your income goes down (or you retire)?
- Who decides how you should enjoy your life (you or an external person)? The answer seems obvious but is worth reiterating for ourselves.
- What role does status and the external image of you and your family play in your expected financial outcomes? This is not a trivial question, and perhaps the most important one for decoupling finances from our life.
- What is the point at which you will accept diminishing or stagnant incomes in exchange for other things in life (including family time, low stress, time for other pursuits, better attention to health and fitness)?
- What parameters, other than income and wealth, do you wish to measure yourself with? This is sometimes harder to come up with, as family time or better health are not always measurable.

Depending on your answers to these questions, you will have to consciously weigh your options or delay the shift to Life 2.0, when the natural tide of things will decide for us. The problem is that, after a point, it may be too late for us to consider Life 2.0 mandates, as old habits die hard. The key characteristic of Life 2.0 is that it affords us sufficient time to reboot and pursue a different agenda from Life 1.0 with different financial goals. Financial goals become a key symbol of our willingness or resistance to move on to Life 2.0. They may further act as a justification for avoiding most of the mandates in this book. This would be a golden opportunity forfeited.

Bestselling author Nassim Nicholas Taleb,[27] who has written books like *The Black Swan* and other popular titles, argues with some wit that, 'The three most harmful addictions are heroin, carbohydrates, and a monthly salary.' He reminds us that we are actually slaves of the steady money that keeps filling our bank accounts.

There is a litmus test to assess your love for money. If you have a second possible source of income (in addition to your principal source) that you can manage simultaneously, would you do the work but forego its income? If you can do this, you have the mental make-up for decoupling finances and life. I recently read about a street vendor who sells wheatgrass juice in Mumbai, India (priced at something like INR 50 per glass). He offers a glass of neem juice—which has several

---

[27]Nassim Nicholas Taleb, https://tinyurl.com/ykdsmsur. Accessed on 4 April 2022.

known natural healing properties, including mitigating diabetes—for free. He could put a price on the neem juice as well but chooses not to. It doesn't cost him anything to get the neem leaves! There is, no doubt, a subtle marketing ploy in this, but the self-restraint against earning additional income is the test of character that I want to highlight here.

Consider this exercise. You are presented with the alternative of a 10 per cent lower income in return for all or some of the following non-monetary experiences and benefits. How would you evaluate them against the monetary sacrifice?

- Two annual vacation periods of 10 days instead of one
- Half a day off every week to look after other needs like caring for elders, etc.
- A 10 per cent raise in your pension
- A seat at the dinner table with an industry icon, held twice a year
- The opportunity to be a keynote speaker at a major charity event that your company participates in
- A week-long, paid family holiday to a place of your choice

The exact arithmetic is not important. It's the principle that matters. Many such trade-offs can be cited. Assess how you would react to them and what alternatives you would prefer. Focus less on the exact value of the options vs the income foregone for this exercise. This is not a hypothetical exercise. In many ways, this is how the income vs other life benefits conundrum plays out in real life. Ernst & Young, the leading accounting and consulting firm, recently introduced for their Australian employees, a 12-week unpaid 'life leave'[28] to travel, do other things or do nothing at all! This may be a harbinger to what the future holds in the life vs work debate. During the 2008 economic recession, countries like Singapore that were highly dependent on global economic activity urged their employers to not retrench employees but pay them less, if necessary. Salary cuts during times of crisis (including the COVID-19 pandemic) are not a new thing. A moderated craving for money helps us prepare for eventualities like these. The farm industry is quite used to this. Incomes from farm produce are seldom stable since the climate, harvest, crop, prices, etc., govern its financial outcomes. These could fluctuate by two to five times for every year (or crop). During and after the pandemic, some salaried people chose to opt out of work for brief periods to stabilize their health or other situations and went back to work, perhaps at another place. This is a forced way to experience and accept varying incomes!

Let us remember that money does not buy everything. It cannot be the only solution to issues like complicated health problems, caring for disabled family members, ruinous habits, etc.

---

[28]'EY introduces up to twelve weeks of unpaid leave for Australian employees', Consultancy.com.au, https://tinyurl.com/mwdhexfd. Accessed on 4 April 2022.

If you are the type of person who likes to chase money because it puts you in some special league of high-net-worth individuals and the fame that comes with it, this section may not be interesting to you. But it may open your eyes to other possibilities that escaped your thoughts. One of the dangerous consequences of not putting brakes on the quest for money is that one may forget that money breeds greed, even if it is a strong word to use. Greed may drive us to improper methods of enhancing income, including bribery, tax avoidance, cheating, trickery, bullying, etc. That is a recipe for dishonesty and unfairness. It only has a beginning and no end.

In this context, it is interesting to analyse Warren Buffett's story. 'I'm already happy. I would be happy, you know—certainly with $100,000 a year, I could be very happy,' Buffett said on PBS NewsHour.[29] At the age of 90, he continues to manage his company, robustly chasing superior financial performances, even though 80 per cent of his wealth (estimated at USD 120 billion) has been pledged to charity.[30] Buffett wishes to maintain his professional success, even though he does not personally enjoy the reward. Consequently, Warren Buffett's legacy is likely to not be just his wealth. This is a case of pursuing financial goals for the sense of accomplishment and experience and

---

[29] Clifford, Catherine. 'Warren Buffett is worth $75 billion but says he would be "very happy" with $100,000 a year', *CNBC Make It*, 12 July 2017, https://tinyurl.com/yckmh44y. Accessed on 4 April 2022.

[30] 'Warren Buffett', The Giving Pledge, https://tinyurl.com/5dx4pmw7. Accessed on 4 April 2022.

not for the direct enjoyment of rewards. Thus, in a sense, it is possible to keep an income goal, a life goal and the pursuit of passion, all in one frame without them colliding.

Many women of my generation (and subsequent ones) face the quandary of pursuing their professional goals while raising their children. Many choose to take a step back from professional pursuits, which has a significant financial implication, to devote time to their life's first priority—their children. Some take a break forever and find it hard to go back to full-time careers. Some women may stay in their careers but opt for a slower track, which obviously brings less income. When it comes to a crunch, how do we choose more sensible options than just money?

You must have noticed the interconnectedness of the ideas in this book. By putting together the last two sections on reassessing our goals and decoupling money and life, we seamlessly reach the next topic—being grateful and gracious. This will, in turn, bring us back to impacting society, learning new skills and other life-changing thoughts. All of these curated thoughts will open the doors to furthering our legacy. The idea of decoupling finances and life may take time to sink in, but it is an important and desirable change in Life 2.0.

Do you wish to challenge yourself on this maxim? Have a true dialogue with your partner and ask each other fundamental questions about your financial status and the trade-offs decoupling your finances and life entails. In Life 2.0, there is a chance to take on this conversation if you reckon you have already achieved your financial goals to a reasonable degree. If you are inclined towards the thought, take the first step—get a job that provides you 25 per cent more time despite its lower income. It may be a tough call, but the proof of this is in the pudding. There will certainly be some withdrawal symptoms—such is the power of money—so, be prepared to stay true to your new belief.

Being Grateful and Gracious

'Gratitude presses outwards and that creates good feelings in the universe. A lot of that comes back to you eventually,' said John Kralik,[31] the author of *365 Thank Yous: The Year a Simple Act of Daily Gratitude Changed My Life*. Kralik made his way out of the extreme pressures of life through daily gratitude notes.

Raymond Zondo, deputy chief justice of the Supreme Court of Appeal of South Africa recently recounted the poignant real-life story[32] of how a local businessman provided free food coupons to his jobless mother and siblings while he was studying law. When the time came to repay that debt, the businessman refused to accept it and instead advised Mr Zondo, 'Just do to others what I have done to you.' This is an extraordinary story of the

---

[31] John Kralik: A Simple Act of Gratitude: How Learning to Say Thank You Changed My Life, https://tinyurl.com/mtrhjj6r. Accessed on 4 April 2022.
[32] Judge Raymond Zondo: A story of Ubuntu that we can all learn from, YouTube, https://tinyurl.com/terc5zs2. Accessed on 4 April 2022.

grateful judge and the gracious businessman. In both cases, this seems like their spontaneous inner response to the situation.

Most of us have a benign attitude towards gratitude and thanking others. We like the idea and the fact that it can create friendly and positive vibes, but we don't practice it as a part of our normal routines. The practice varies according to cultures too. If we prepare a list of things that we need to thank the creator (or someone else) for, it would run into a long list. There are many things that we know or can do that are taken for granted. How do we acknowledge our gratitude for these and how often?

In meditation routines, one of the first activities is gratitude meditation. You are asked to set aside all other thoughts and spend about 10 minutes thanking a lot of things and people. You start with your body and organs, without which you can't exist—there are at least a hundred known organs that we need to thank (and this just includes the more common ones, not the various glands in our body or the processors in the respiratory or digestive systems) for helping us live our daily lives. We think of the little finger only when it hurts or we cut or burn it. Our neck gets attention when we have an awkward sprain. Similarly, our knee gets attention in our fifties or sixties, when it refuses to perform its normal functions, and so on. It seems formal and bizarre to thank our organs, but if you imagine for a moment how you would not be able to function normally if even one of them breaks down, you realize their importance better. We will understand the significance of each organ better when we see others who cannot perform simple physical activities that we are able to. Thanking our organs formally is a good way to recognize their vital contribution to our daily lives.

The gratitude mindset has a prerequisite—being able to focus on the things we have and have had rather than the ones we have missed (or the things that others have). It is a classic case of glass half-full or half-empty. All the things that we have and enjoy in life belong to a similar category of what life gives us, but we are not consciously grateful for any for them. Do we have a good family life? Do we have the right kind of friends? Do we have optimal material comforts? Do we live in a home that we like? Have we had a satisfactory career? Did we achieve our educational goals? Have we lived free of major health issues? Do we sleep well (most of the time)? Do we get to eat the kind of food we like on most days? These are just sample questions. You probably answered 'yes' to many of these questions but most likely don't think that there are some people who are playing a part in getting us these things. Who are they and do we thank them, even by remembering them?

Stacking up our needs according to Maslow's hierarchy,[33] and ticking off the needs that are being met substantially or fully is another way to draw up a 'thanking list'. Apart from any meditation routine, many of us pray to thank

---

[33] McLeod, Saul. 'Maslow's Hierarchy of Needs', SimplyPsychology, 2007, https://tinyurl.com/y2buhbfn. Accessed on 4 April 2022.

our favourite god. Some people donate money or other expensive objects to the Almighty. Some do it in more socially useful ways like building schools, feeding the poor or offering them health services for free. These are surrogate ways of expressing our gratitude to the Almighty for what we enjoy. Unfortunately, the number of people practising gratitude is relatively small. Most of us do not thank god by serving his creation or thank people who help us succeed.

Thanking is easy but significant...

> *The roots of all goodness lie in the soil of appreciation for goodness.*
>
> —The Dalai Lama

What is a good way to offer our gratitude to the countless things we have and those who have supported us? It could be in our own style and suitable to our own methods. We could start with a simple 'thank you'. Saying thanks 10 or 20 times a day to various people or organizations, verbally, through phone messages or emails is a good start. It gets us into the habit and keeps prodding us not to miss the occasions to practise gratitude. More grateful gestures could take the form of physically or financially assisting someone in need, thanksgiving prayers and appreciation records. Some prefer to give people thank you cards for any act of help or kindness. Making the expression of our gratitude regular and prolific will develop a subconscious habit, almost like greeting someone when you meet a person for the first time on a day.

There is another way to be thankful indirectly—stop complaining about things that do not go our way, which can include our daily food, the traffic, our co-workers' actions, the weather, the cost of certain items that we buy or consume, etc. If we reflect on these things carefully, we will realize that when they were all going our way, we never thanked anyone for them. So, we do not have a 'thanks bank' to borrow from when things flip around, to our chagrin. I have even seen some people who would find fault with their parents for not doing something for them when they were younger. Just pause to think what all they have done to help you become a confident citizen. Parents have to often exercise some judgment, evaluate trade-offs and work within their constraints—financial or otherwise. Considering these, most of our parents did their best for their children without holding anything back. However, we take all this for granted. The next time you have a complaint, think of all the things that had gone right until that moment.

Thanking or expressing gratitude has another positive side effect of reminding us how privileged we are compared to many others in society. Thus, the act of thanking is a good leveller. We also have to reflect on the phenomenon of being dissatisfied, even when we get something. We may still regret that we could have gotten something better. I certainly thought so after I got my Joint Entrance Examination rank to be admitted into the Indian Institute of Technology (IIT), which wasn't great! Thanks are due irrespective of whether you make it. The thanking routine puts things in a better perspective because it reminds you that you could have been worse off (and fortunately, you aren't). When you are content with something and, therefore, thankful, you perhaps would be less obsessed with wanting more or better things. It could activate the thought that outcomes have a tendency of finding their fair levels.

Psychologists suggest maintaining a 'gratitude journal' to record at least one thing every day for which you are grateful and list who you are grateful to for it. Over time, this does not just become a journal but a transformational tool for reflection. In the previous generations, thoughts and experiences were largely stored in the mind. With increased longevity and the prospect of memory loss in the later stages of life, it has become a necessity to write our stories and reflections. It's also a good new habit to cultivate.

A lot of research has also been done linking the act of gratitude to its psychological effects on those who practise it. Neuroscientists have proved that extending gratitude generates neurotransmitters like dopamine, which makes us feel good, and serotonin, which enhances our mood and acts as a kind of antidepressant. These neurotransmitters are released by our neural circuitry when we offer gratitude and reflect on the positives.[34] So, we gain two things by being

---

[34]Burton, Linda Roszak. 'The Neuroscience of Gratitude: What you need to know about the new neural knowledge'. *Wharton Alumni Club: University of Pennsylvania*, https://tinyurl.com/3u5tvyd8. Accessed on 4 April 2022.

grateful—appreciation of each act in our present and our legacy for our afterlife.

Graciousness, in some ways, is on the same spectrum of expression as gratitude, but it is subtly different. It is the act of not just being grateful but practising forgiveness, being magnanimous and giving up on something for another person, either as a sacrifice or out of deference. You are considered gracious if you give up your right to the last remaining seat on a plane to help a sick person who needs to travel more urgently than you. This is gracious because you do not need to give up your right. Similarly, thanking your former boss for all that you are achieving in your professional career is graciousness because you don't have to do it. Perhaps he is not even remotely responsible for your success, but thanking him would certainly make him happy. Not all acts of kindness are classifiable as gracious. The gesture has to be voluntary and out of the ordinary for it to be considered gracious. Through both gratefulness and graciousness, we display a certain tenderness in us that is considered one of the hallmarks of a good leader.

In an excerpt from the book *Why Forgive?*, author Johann Christoph Arnold narrates the story of Steven McDonald, a young police officer who was shot by a teenager in New York's Central Park in 1986, which left him paralysed. 'I forgave [the shooter] because I believe the only thing worse than receiving a bullet in my spine would have been to nurture revenge in my heart,' McDonald wrote.[35] While the younger man was serving his prison sentence, McDonald corresponded with him, hoping that one day the two could work together to demonstrate forgiveness and non-violence. This is an exemplary case of forgiveness in the face of severe personal adversity. We get many chances to do something similar, even if we haven't suffered as much, and all those chances count.

One would think that graciousness would be an inherent trait among humans. Sadly, for far too long, society has peddled on individual goals, often in competition with others. Otherwise, why would we need signs in commuter trains assigning corner seats to people with disabilities, pregnant people and those in need of physical help? That should be the default human response anyway! However, we have reached a point where we need explicit reminders to be gracious, even in the most obvious situations.

It is useful to analyse the curious case of graciousness (or lack thereof) among colleagues at work or in a public setting. Graciousness has no direct benefit except for pleasing, creating goodwill or having a feel-good effect on another person without you losing much. However, by doing this, a silent stash of credit grows in your account. In the Hindu tradition, this is believed to be another form of good karma that will have a payback in another world or life. However, one often finds that people are unwilling to cede credit to

---

[35] Arnold, Johann Christoph. *Why Forgive*, Orbis Books, 30 November 2009.

colleagues where due.

Writing for *The New York Times*, renowned columnist David Brooks says,

> If you treat the world as a friendly and hopeful place, as a web of relationships, you'll look for the good news in people and not the bad. You'll be willing to relinquish control, and in surrender you'll actually gain more strength as people trust in your candour and come alongside. Gracious leaders create a more gracious environment by greeting the world openly and so end up maximizing their influence and effectiveness.[36]

Perhaps the epitome of being gracious was Nobel laureate and South African President Nelson Mandela famously remarking, 'Forget the past,' even as he got out of prison after being locked up for 27 years for a crime he hadn't committed. What would have been his mental frame when he said it?

There is a reason for bringing both gratitude and graciousness into this book. Not everyone has these qualities by default. In a competitive and materialistic world, practising these qualities is considered difficult, as progress of the self is often the goal in Life 1.0. However, Life 2.0 is a good reflection point to first question, and then change our habits and attitudes, if we have not practised either of these well or at all. It is also an opportunity to

---

[36]Brooks, David. 'The Art of Gracious Leadership', *The New York Times*, 26 August 2016, https://tinyurl.com/y8sezs6k. Accessed on 4 April 2022.

set right an adverse or neutral legacy when it comes to good behaviour. As mentioned earlier, these niceties are not always in our armoury when we are chasing the goals that matter to our fortune and status more than the ones that kindle our soul. In fact, we often work against kindling our souls when we are young and striving to steady our lives and careers. We tend to be so competitive that we practise the opposite of graciousness—meanness! We tend to do this when we are focused on achieving the material goals of life. This is easily explained by the concept of sportsmanship in competitive sports.

Legendary Argentinian footballer Diego Maradona, who passed away in 2020, had his moment of glory when he scored a goal for Argentina in the 1986 Football World Cup final that won his country the coveted cup. It was later discovered that he may have used his hand to score the goal. But he did not claim his winning shot in the fifty-first minute of the final against England as a hand-goal because that would not have won the gold medal for Argentina and permanent fame for himself. On the other hand, a member of the Cyprus Canoe Federation and the Limassol Nautical Club, Christiana Pavlou, was first in the national ranking for her category of 15-year-olds. On 25 September 2012, at the Cyprus Canoe Sprint National Championship in Limassol, she participated in the K2 200-metre event and won the competition. However, after the race, she went to the race officials and told them that her team had, in fact, crossed the finish line second and not first. Consequently, she

THE MANDATES: COORDINATES OF A NEW JOURNEY 91

deliberately deprived herself of the title. She was only 15 then! Even if Christiana wasn't as successful in her later endeavours as she might have wanted to be, she achieved the important goal of keeping a clear conscience for the rest of her life and a laudable legacy. When such a moment stares at you, what is your instinctive response? Many sports have now brought in fair play awards to encourage a groundswell of better on-field rectitude.[37] There is also the recent story of an Italian defender, 17-year-old Mattia Agnese, who instinctively administered first-aid to an opponent who had suffered a concussion and had stopped breathing. Agnese won the FIFA fair play award in 2020. What do these youngsters have in common? They have a gracious streak by default. There are other famous role models of such graciousness, like Indian cricketers Rahul Dravid and Anil Kumble, and tennis legend Roger Federer. These are people at the highest level of their fields who have not only played fairly but also espoused graciousness as their second nature. If it is not your second nature, perhaps you need to reflect and bring it into your routine, and Life 2.0 offers you the opportunity to do so.

When my career took a dramatic turn and moved me to the sales function (from accounting) at the start of my second professional decade, my daily routine at work changed, as you would imagine. I was meeting a large number of business-to-business (B2B) customers, most of whom were helping our business progress either directly

---

[37]International Fair Play Committee, https://tinyurl.com/32s9ns53. Accessed on 4 April 2022.

or indirectly. Several small acts or gestures of gratitude and graciousness moved the needle in our favour. This triggered in me the skill and consciousness to say 'thanks' much more than I had done before (accountants do need a lot of EQ!). I did not want to make it seem like our B2B clients' actions were a quid pro quo. Hence, I consciously developed gratitude into a routine. It seems simple, but the transformation was harder than one would think. Learning to say thanks genuinely and spontaneously is not easy. I had to remind myself when the occasions arose. This awareness also develops with practice. One trick is to say it several times a day, even for small things. If done well, the receiver will notice it and you will get your quota of practice. Equanimity in success and defeat is another variant of graciousness, as is giving credit where it is due.

I was a recipient of surprise graciousness once in my early work life. As a young manager in my twenties, I was meeting my divisional director and his boss, the executive director of the company, about a task. At the start of the meeting, my divisional director introduced me and said, 'He has just earned a creditable promotion.' I was too stumped and embarrassed to even say thanks because my mind was reminding me that those were the two people who had approved my promotion, and yet, they were generous enough to give me credit!

Another such eye-opening conversation happened with one of the cleaners of my condominium who was leaving her job to take up another one. The lady had passed through several misfortunes and setbacks in her life with her children, and yet, she was at the workplace promptly at 7.00 a.m. every day, doing her duties diligently and always with a smile. She motivated herself and never really received any greetings from others. From that day, I have made it a practice to greet the cleaners every day, engaging in a short conversation with them and thanking them for keeping our environment clean and hygienic. To me, that lady was going beyond her circumstances to be gracious, and I needed to be more grateful to her and people like her. It was a sort of awakening that I wish I had had much earlier. It's something that comes naturally to my wife.

Besides our competitive nature and our selfish interests, there are other factors that stifle our propensity for graciousness. These factors include the fact that graciousness has no clear rewards in the conventional sense, brings no publicity or fame, may be misinterpreted as weakness and is a one-way street. Once you are firmly on the path to graciousness, you will keep to it, which could, sometimes, be exploited by others. For example, if you give up your place in a queue, some undeserving people may jump ahead of you. Being gracious is also sometimes considered defeatist. You can't be selectively gracious, as you would attract the criticism of being biased. By being gracious, you often postpone gratification and a sense of achievement in your activities.

With so much against it, why should we be gracious? The answer lies within us. It is for self-enjoyment and for satiating the heart and soul. If Life 2.0 is about evolving ourselves as human beings who are sharing the planet, we can see the reasons clearly. Graciousness is often equated with kindness, grace, compassion, sacrifice, thoughtfulness, empathy, tact, restraint, spontaneity, blessing and even acceptance (physically or metaphorically). Many religions have the notion that those who are gracious are touched or blessed by god. The phrase 'goodness gracious' is not without a foundation. The absence of harsh words and unfriendly deeds or gestures in our lives is considered equally gracious. In Christianity, there is the notion that we must walk (carry ourselves) lightly on earth. That is a call to be gentle and compassionate. In Hinduism, Mother Earth is a goddess, who should be worshipped and not exploited, along with her creations. Graciousness is infectious and can transfer from your associates and family members to you or vice versa. Teachers are often trained and exhorted to exemplify graciousness so that children can learn it through observation when they are young.

Like the other topics discussed earlier in this book, gratitude is also entirely optional. Each of us must convince ourselves of what it could do for us, our personality, our legacy or our identity in society. The reward is purely internal satisfaction, leading to self-actualization. Furthermore, such rewards come when we consistently practise the trait and not just on the odd occasion. So, once again, the trigger is with us. How do we begin to make the changes?

THE MANDATES: COORDINATES OF A NEW JOURNEY

Changing our behaviour to be grateful and gracious

> *It is not right to forget the help rendered by*
> *someone; it is virtuous to forget any harm,*
> *the moment it is done.*

—Chapter 11, Righteousness Part, *Thirukkural*[38]

If expressing gratitude is not one of our current virtues, we could do some or all of the following activities to embrace it consciously:

- Say thanks to 10 people every day (verbally or in writing).
- Be considerate to people who need assistance in bus, train or bank queues. Stand aside and let them go ahead.
- Give credit to a spouse or child for some good thing that happened at home.
- Give credit to a colleague for an achievement at work. Better still, say it publicly.
- Share an award or reward with your teammates.
- Avoid pointing out someone's mistake if it does not matter (this is my wife's advice to me).
- Postpone criticism—you may decide against your comment later or find better words to put it.
- Praise an achievement of a colleague or a family

---

[38] Thiruvalluvar. *Thirukkural*, G.U. Pope (trans.), Createspace Independent Publishing Platform, 31 August 2017.

member, even if you have contributed significantly to that achievement.
- Be patient.
- Recall any person who helped you in the past and write an appreciation note, even if a long time has passed since they helped you.
- Do a gratitude prayer.
- Talk less and listen more (this itself is an act of gracious deference).
- Disagree without being disagreeable.
- Offer to forego your entitlement (may be the prize money in a lottery), if you think someone else could benefit more from it.
- Welcome a friend who you may have parted from with some bitterness back into your life.
- Take time to thank a former boss for how well you are doing in your career or life, some of which may be due to his or her guidance.
- Think before speaking. Say the appropriate thing.
- Ask for forgiveness if you have made a mistake, even if no one has lost anything. It's good to remind ourselves of our own missteps.
- Be careful with words (and tone) in written communication. We can often come across as ungracious, even if our intentions are not such.
- Keep a diary of incidents listing the missed opportunities to be gracious or grateful.
- Ask for feedback on your behaviour and receive it sincerely and well.

- Show humility and don't flaunt success.
- Be the person you want others to be in every transaction.
- Have friendlier body language while communicating (this may be hard for those who never bothered about it before).
- Cultivate a lower sense of entitlement (this can be difficult for some).
- If you are the bean-counter type, keep a record of all the moments when you were overly inconsiderate and use it to measure your progress towards having a better demeanour.

Well, that's a long laundry list, and yet, it may not seem complete! Even if we practise a few of these things consciously, we could get into a virtuous cycle. You would also observe that being grateful or gracious have very limited downsides in the form of losses—financial or otherwise. No loss and some gain is clearly a compelling duty call. You also don't need to find any special resource or embrace other compromises. Of all the commandments (mandates) in this book, this is the easiest to begin!

Sharing and Coaching

Knowledge shared is power multiplied.
—Robert Noyce, Co-Founder, Intel

We all fondly reminisce about a few kind teachers from our school and college days, long after our student years. Many such teachers impact us, our beliefs, characters and choices. They leave their indelible mark on our minds. They may not have actually planned to secure a legacy but receive it automatically. There is something noble about sharing selflessly and out of free will. I salute the readers who are professional teachers. For the rest of us, though, the teaching moment comes later in life in a different form, as we will discuss in this section.

We are learners all our lives. Formal learning at schools and colleges gives way to informal education during our career, family life and exposure to the world and new experiences. We store all this learning without quite thinking about its future uses. The beauty of such learning is that many of the new learnings raise their head at appropriate times to shore up our ability to manage new challenges. Conflict resolution is a case in point. Young people have limited skills for this because they have not developed the nuances in communication, judgement and perspective that are necessary for it. Experience brings heightened skill levels and new tools that we can use. You would realize that you manage the same conflict differently in your mid-forties as compared to your early twenties. You may even walk away with better outcomes, despite employing softer tactics, or perhaps because of them.

All of us have had to muster old learnings and add new learnings to cope with the crisis of the COVID-19 pandemic.

THE MANDATES: COORDINATES OF A NEW JOURNEY 99

This crisis impacted various aspects of our lives, including education, work, family, health, finances and relationships. Many would confirm that their skill sets improved during this period that saw us fight for our survival.

Professor Indira Parikh, a long-time faculty at my alma mater, the Indian Institute of Management, Ahmedabad, and an authority on organizational development and personal growth says that knowledge is complete only with experiences. According to her, 'seeing the invisible and hearing the inaudible,'[39] are essential to a complete learning process. Therefore, learning (and simultaneously, teaching or coaching) is a lifelong pursuit. As long as there are good learners, good teachers (who can be seen as sharers) are necessary. This is the origin of the sharing philosophy outlined in this section.

The knowledge, skills and experiences that we keep accumulating are like books in our private library. If we catalogue them, they could amount to a sizable possession. What are the different ways in which we can use these assets? How would we want our library (of ideas, skills, talent) to be shared or used by others after our lives are over (or even while we live)? Unfortunately, this thought does not occur to us in the normal course of our lives.

I strongly believe that we are all teachers of some kind too. The instructional instinct is sometimes latent until a later stage in life. Life 2.0 is one possible point to revive it.

---

[39] World HRD Congress 2018 - PROF. INDIRA PARIKH, YouTube, https://tinyurl.com/yn3h7a52. Accessed on 4 April 2022.

The accumulated expertise, knowledge and situational skills acquired while navigating Life 1.0 have great potential to be deployed on others and by others. Some people take to formal teaching (as many of my management classmates and I did), while others find similar avenues like corporate training, mentoring (sometimes pro bono), lecturing, etc. At the least, we try to coach our children, nephews, nieces, and other next generation kids in the neighbourhood. Professional teaching requires formal exposure to teaching methods, pastoral and motivational styles, mechanics, appropriate communication and other skills unique to the profession. It is surprising that the several years of career and life experiences teach us most of these as well. Thus, we are able to switch to the coaching or teaching mode almost unnoticed, should the opportunity present itself.

The famous American poet and playwright, Robert Frost (1874–1963) said, 'I am not a teacher; I am an awakener.' The reference to awakening here is significant, as it confirms that people just need someone to trigger an unearthing of knowledge and emotions that reside within everyone. Helping others succeed is an allied thought in this context. There are many people who are not only unsuccessful but are resigned to not try. This view of life robs them of their dreams and leaves them helpless, with no goals. They badly need someone to lift their spirits, help them set realistic goals and trigger action. This is similar to sharing knowledge or coaching.

A friend of mine has taken coaching to be her lifelong pursuit, neither for money nor professionally but as a full-time hobby. She champions issues like sustainability, water conservation, youth leadership, social awareness in the digital world, etc. Her modus operandi is to work with groups of young people in schools or outside them, initiating projects that provide them experiences in these areas, instead of classroom teaching or reading from a book. She is almost a crusader for imparting these sensitivities to young minds. This is the perfect example of coaching (and transferring what we know) to another generation, with clear outcomes in mind. These initiatives are not without the usual hurdles such as lack of time, difficulty in generating the required enthusiasm, lack of resources, sustainability of efforts, etc. Despite facing all these issues, every morning, my friend's determination is higher than the previous day!

Famous sports personalities have tended to offer their coaching services for free to community youth, especially in low-income societies. Rafael Nadal from Spain and Michael Johnson from the US are perfect examples. Olympic legend Michael Johnson brought young leaders from 10 different countries together for a week-long summit at his cutting-edge performance centre in Texas, furthering his support of young people by working, leading and improving their community through sports. This was done through the Michael Johnson Foundation.[40] This programme aims to

---

[40]'Michael Johnson Convenes Young Leaders in Dallas Summit', Coaches Across Continents, https://tinyurl.com/33kvbhj9. Accessed on 4 April 2022.

develop a sporting culture and build youth leaders who will serve their communities with superior skills honed by world-renowned athletes. The cherry on the cake is that this programme is fully sponsored. Michael Johnson took this up early in what could be considered his Life 2.0, after his days as an active player.

Harry M. Kraemer has achieved another such unique feat. He was the CEO of Baxter International Inc., a healthcare company worth USD 12 billion dollar.[41] In his Life 2.0, he became one of the revered strategy professors at the prestigious Kellogg School of Management, Northwestern University, USA. He went on to win the best professor of the year award at the university in 2008 and wrote a couple of bestsellers. His is a story of a stunning switch to teaching and sharing, even if one acknowledges that his teaching is a commercial assignment.

My baby steps towards sharing my experience and knowledge started at work. I began training my own colleagues and teams on subjects like account management, communication, negotiation, selling skills, creativity, etc. Those initial forays gave me the confidence and experience to scale up later. When Life 2.0 arrived (around 2006, according to my reckoning), I had more time to devote towards formal, university-level teaching, albeit on a part-time basis. Thanks to some common contacts of my brother, who is an academic, I landed my first undergraduate

---

[41] 'Harry M. Kraemer', Northwestern Kellogg, https://tinyurl.com/3utrr7z5. Accessed on 4 April 2022.

teaching contract for a full course instantly. I started to enjoy the experience immensely (the monetary gain was nothing to write home about) and went on to teach other courses, and at other universities, for nearly a decade. My stint extended to being a project coach for an executive education programme that my university ran for a leading global technology and consulting company. This opportunity offered me new avenues of learning and skill deployment because my students were senior managers, some as old as me, with over 20 years of working experience. This task was more in the nature of sharing, coaching and guiding, and required slightly different skills and approach. If someone had asked me 20 years ago whether I would ever teach at university level, I would have called it a joke. But circumstances change and so do the manifestation of our latent abilities and interests.

My undergraduate teaching and executive coaching experiences had their own distinct challenges. These experiences brought me into a virtuous cycle of learning further on the job and teaching me new skills and tools along the way. I paused after nearly 10 years of teaching to focus my attention on my business interests. At the K-12 school that I helped co-found, I run short workshops on communication, productivity, leadership, etc. It's a good feeling to try and help others become lifelong learners. Such activities are now an important passion for me and have dovetailed into my new vocations of teaching and writing.

Writing is sharing too...

> *Share your knowledge. It's a way to achieve immortality.*
>
> —The Dalai Lama

We see people who resort to a more passive way of sharing—writing! When we write an article or a book, fiction or non-fiction, we are sharing our ideas, knowledge, coherent narration, linguistic facets, moods, thoughts, questions, answers, logic, emotions, hypotheses, facts, opinions, writing styles, facets of our personality, biases, likes and beliefs. The lens through which we see the world, the happenings around us and the events in our lives, are visible and useful lessons that a writer learns. This is a beautiful way to transfer one's learning and experiences to a large group of readers who willingly read and enjoy the work. Each reader takes up the responsibility to learn from his or her reading of all that has been shared by the writer. Thus, a book or an article is a reservoir through which a writer can share myriad things. Mahatma Gandhi, Nelson Mandela and Martin Luther King may not have taught but their lessons are spread across their conversations about leadership, life choices, kindness, humility, humanity, etc. Many writers have even influenced revolutions by subtly impacting thoughts and minds through a certain form of storytelling that draws on our senses. Thus, writers are teachers too.

As an extension of my teaching and coaching interests,

I have authored a book on B2B account management based on my corporate sales experience. Published in 2018, the book intends to be a practical guide for those who see themselves in the jobs that I was doing. Again, the writing experience was different from just knowing the subject. The imperative for authors is that they ponder, organize their thoughts, put themselves in the readers' shoes, bring out expert insights, intersperse ideas and examples while using simple language and narration. This book on Life 2.0 has taken me in a new direction as well because its contents are more universal and personally relatable. I also published a book on habits for smart skill-building in 2021 where I discussed my thoughts on another favourite topic—lifelong learning.[42] This is a livelier way of sharing one's experiences and creative thoughts. One of my colleagues at the university where I taught once said to me, 'If I want to learn a new subject, I offer to teach it!' This is a profound observation. You will need to acquire a certain degree of thoroughness in a subject before you can impart any kind of learning. This sets you on a learning path. The commitment to teach triggers the action required to learn the subject. Those who buy a lot of self-improvement or other similar books know the ills of not reading them conscientiously or of the subsequent lethargy that sets in while applying the ideas. Imagine if you had to read a book and conduct a workshop for others based on that book. What would your degree of

---

[42]Shankar, Bala. *The Twelve Habits of Smart Skill-Building: A Code for the Reskilling of You*, Penguin Random House SEA, 27 September 2021.

interest in the contents of the book have to be for you to be able to share your insights and inferences usefully? To implement this idea in the educational institution that I co-founded, it is a standard practice for teachers to deliver a training session to their colleagues based on their own learning from an external training programme that they attend.

Learn further to teach better

This brings us to the interesting phenomenon of coaches perhaps having a selfish motive to hone their abilities. When you teach or guide someone even informally, you start becoming more adept at doing it. Even when you help a child assemble a toy, you are learning to do it. So, teaching or coaching is in our interest for yet another reason, besides our legacy and social usefulness. Some of the courses I taught forced me to study more intensely about the nuances and the practice of the topic at hand, even if I was familiar with the general concepts. I re-entered a professional library after many decades as I prepared to teach full courses! As late-stage learning is tougher, teaching a subject can be a good resilience test and can raise our productivity. The concepts we learn are also put to test as we need to gain the confidence of the students we teach. In most universities now, the faculty are rated by students, and these ratings are published (so, it's not enough to just get by!). In fact, students' feedback is one of the important criteria for faculty reappointment. When I started to write my account management book, I realized that the conceptual frameworks that led to my moments of success needed to be crafted in such a way that they guide the readers. That led me back to the literature, stepping up my reading on the subject and its adjacencies. I am very grateful for the push the writing project gave me.

In Life 2.0, we have the opportunity to be useful to others by transferring our knowledge more than casually. 'Teach a man to fish rather than give him fish' is a famous saying. Instead of our doing things for others, we could help them learn how to do them themselves. Pro bono coaching or mentoring has another unseen advantage. It could start a new paid opportunity stream for you, if satisfied students refer you to other clients. This is an inexpensive way to build your testimonials. Reid Hoffman, the founder of LinkedIn, refers to this in his popular book, *The Start-up of You*, in the context of reskilling for new careers or jobs.

Sharing has won spiritual backing too. There is a famous quote by the Buddha that exhorts man to selflessly share, 'Thousands of candles can be lighted from a single candle, and the life of the candle will not be shortened. Happiness never reduces by being shared.'

This quote has a subtle message that a candle does not derive any personal advantage in the process of lighting many more.

One of my daughter's employers, a US multinational, has a system of reverse-mentoring. In this activity, younger employees coach and mentor the older or senior employees in modern-day technologies, digital literacy and the new media landscape. It is a weekly or monthly calendared activity and is monitored by the human resources team. While the purpose is clear, the novelty of getting younger employees involved in this activity engages them more in organizational learning, helps them get to know the different cadres of employees and is an early baptism in coaching. Additionally, it nudges senior employees to be humble students when the situation demands.

So, how does one start teaching or coaching? Everyone may not reckon that he or she is a good teacher or coach. The reality is that it does not matter. This is something that can be adapted to your proven capabilities. There are several coaching styles, and one can, with some effort, fit into one of those styles.

The who, what and when?

Remember that when you leave this earth, you can take with you nothing that you have received—only what you have given.

—St. Francis of Assisi

The first premise for embracing the mandate of sharing and coaching is deciding the who, what and when of it. The how will follow.

Who? Who are the people that you reckon would benefit from your sharing or coaching? Pick the profiles and groups that you will enjoy coaching, and who will reciprocate your enthusiasm. Since it has no clear rewards, the experience of coaching must be enjoyable and satisfying in itself. This depends a lot on the group dynamics and the working relationship of the coach with the coached. One criterion is the age group. Would you rather coach adults than teenagers? Often, coaching strangers is easier than coaching familiar people. Another dimension to consider is whether the coached are self-learners or need hand-holding. Students, colleagues, social groups, walking buddies, drinking enthusiasts, apartment neighbours, readers' clubs, dog walkers' groups, service groups in temples or churches—there are many groups to choose from. It is now possible to target pupil groups based on their social media behaviour or topics of interest. You will be surprised as to how many unserved groups exist with people who need a specific coach for something and cannot find one (or the right one).

What? What are some areas that we think we have some unique skills or expertise in? Stick to your areas of competence since that would make the take-off smooth. It is good to take a sequential approach to it, as a teacher would. For example, if you wish to coach young graduates on career choices, start by understanding their desires, aptitudes and abilities. Matching choices to individual needs helps the mentee relate to the prescriptions better. Choose a sustainable topic that goes beyond an initiation or a one-off engagement. One of my friends decided to offer an appreciation course on classical music. Not everyone has the basic orientation for this. He began at such a high level that the group was intimidated away quickly. Similarly, the group members need to have the right motivation to get coached—financial rewards are not enough. There has to be an intrinsic desire. You may also need to decide on different segments of an overall topic or area so that your efforts can be aligned to previous segments. For example, if you choose an area like spoken English for frontline sales staff (obviously for non-native speakers), you need to plan a few cascading levels in order to cater to fast and slow learners in the same group. So, focus on what needs careful planning. You may even need lesson plans!

When? How much time can we spare for our coaching activity and how often? To ensure a good and sustainable level of commitment, we need to be realistic about the amount of time we are willing to 'sacrifice'. A half-hearted effort with erratic time allocation will fail. For instance, if we are coaching senior citizens in basic smartphone usage, can we dedicate a certain number of hours per week for a set period of time? Please remember that even if it is pro bono, and out of genuine interest, you will still desire some outcome, such as improvements in the level of skill of the person being taught. This requires an honest allocation of time. With digital avenues springing up, it is now possible to conduct virtual sessions. Another friend of mine taught the Valmiki Ramayana (the highly revered original Sanskrit text of the popular Indian epic, Ramayana) to a group of learners (mostly young) located in different continents via Skype, at a particular time and day every week. He sustained it for over 50 weeks and brought it to a logical end, including a finale! Caring for the participants' time preferences is also important, especially if the topic is non-vocational or out of special interest.

Once the above factors are in place, it is easy to fit in the 'how'. What forms of sharing will suit your group? It could be webinars, closed-door sessions, online sessions, chat forums, classroom lectures, group activities followed by summary discussions, one-to-one conversations, podcasts, audio books, question-answer interactions, as is often done in spiritual journeys, readings followed by clarifying dialogues, etc. One size does not fit all! Some trial and error may be necessary if you are teaching or coaching for the first time. The 'what' and the 'how' will sustain the interest of the ones under your tutelage. Like all pursuits, the first taste of success takes time, but the subsequent ones are yours to reap. Given the free nature of such sessions, it is possible that the participants will alternate between high and low interest from time to time. It is, therefore, critical to follow a progressive approach, which means that those who struggle to keep up should not be left behind.

Sharing can also happen through talks, speaking roles in public forums, panel participation and the like. People with a public profile tend to prefer this mode as it economizes their time. Such forms of sharing have a good reach but are often one-off and low-intensity activities. Besides, they do not help establish a sustained rapport with the participants that may be the key to real transfer of skills or knowledge. Talks and lectures are meant to share nuggets of knowledge or to inspire participants to get involved more.

Coaching is an important leadership trait that is formally included in appraisals of senior managers in the corporate world. Your success depends on the success of the people who work for you, and it becomes your duty to equip them with the knowledge and skills that will help them perform. In the modern world, coaching is also considered a therapy, one that takes the mind away from other anxieties and contexts. I haven't experienced it personally, but there is a good possibility that it does. Writing is also sharing. Blogs are the new tool for sharing, especially since reading is a reasonably effective way of learning. It could be a starting point for people who are shy conversationalists. However, writing does not assure sustained contact. Two-way online forums yield better results in terms of visible engagement and transfer.

Life 2.0 is an opportunity to share our stored knowledge or special abilities. Don't wait a moment. Choose a group and a topic, and experience this wonderful journey. There is a teacher in every one of us, and there is knowledge to be shared. There is no better way to create a club of grateful learners and beneficiaries who will hopefully add an important chapter to your legacy script.

Reshaping Communication

A man's character may be learned from the adjectives which he habitually uses in conversations.

—Mark Twain

I have a senior friend, about 30 years older, who is a highly successful lawyer and a former parliamentarian, bred in British decorum and a practitioner of the grammar of gentlemanliness. I invited him to an event, and he consented but had to withdraw due to another important event. Besides asking his secretary to send his apologies the day before the event, he called me on the day of the event and said, 'Bala, I must start off with an apology...' He didn't need to call a person 30 years his junior (and by any measure, a much less accomplished one) nor did he have to apologize twice, including over a phone call. It just happens to be the DNA of his communication etiquette. He has practised it for 60–70 years and perfected it over time. This is his default code.

Civilization has seen many significant changes in communication strategies, methods and modes that have shaped narratives, conversations and sensibilities, leading to the evolution of its nuances. Kautilya, the famous statecraft expert of India, said, 'Purity of speech, of the mind, of the senses, and of a compassionate heart are needed by one who desires to rise to the divine platform.'[43]

The fact that he puts the onus of a higher order communication on the self is quite interesting because, often, the opposite is true. It is human nature to blame any failures in communication or poor communication on the receivers!

If there is one thing that offers lifelong learning, it is communication—oral, written and even body language. It can never be perfect. Our approach to communication as youngsters is more direct, to the point and even brash or offensive. Kind or polite words don't make it to our vocabulary at that stage. Our frame of mind is fully reflected in what we say or what we write (no double guessing is considered necessary at this age). As youngsters, we believe that the rest of the world should be able to understand why we communicate in a certain way. Very often, we are not even aware of the consequences of our style of communication. When I was a young executive (as an accountant), the only way I knew to say 'no' was to say just that word—I had no nuanced way to put it. If anything, my body language accentuated its harshness.

Thankfully, refinements do come in at every stage. How do we improve this skill over the years? For some, there is little change, and the brashness continues to various degrees. There may also be an ego factor in communication that conditions some to be dominant (in a negative sense),

---

[43] Mark, Joshua. 'Arthashastra', *World History Encyclopedia*, 23 June 2020, https://tinyurl.com/5n79yxwe. Accessed on 4 April 2022.

offensive, sarcastic, condescending and even alienating. The more it is practised, the more it gets ingrained as part of one's personality. It may even become a permanent feature for some. Fortunately, it is possible to correct this tendency with proper intervention at an early stage.

As we grow older, we realize that it is not enough to focus merely on the message. Our focus shifts from the message to its tone and language, from the speaker/writer to the receiver, from effectiveness to a holistic outcome, from standard to customized messaging and from mechanical to emotional content. Every communication can be used as a tool to enhance relationships and reflect positivity. If it is not used properly, it can lead to the opposite effect too!

Age and experience bring in refinements in our personality and communication. I strongly believe in this, especially for non-native speakers. Our operating vocabulary is enhanced with subtler and more nuanced words. For example, we stop saying 'I don't like it' (in the context of food). Instead, we begin to say, 'My taste preference is a little different,' which is a smoother, less offensive way of saying the same thing. Our tone and use of emotively powerful words begin to reflect some sensitivity to the listener of the message. The listener forms a composite understanding of the message from all the elements of communication. He or she understands the subtleties of language, but the main meaning is never sacrificed.

Since the enhancements in communication happen in a natural process, we don't necessarily measure the progress or the effectiveness. We may be unaware of the further refinements that are needed. This is because communication is seen as a natural phenomenon and not one that could be shaped significantly by intervention. This is, however, a wrong notion. We let the passage of time take care of the improvements. That may or may not be enough (it may be too late or too little). Therefore, a more conscious stocktaking and remediation becomes necessary to make our communication effective and well-modulated.

There is adequate evidence that in public life (and in corporate careers and spiritual spheres), communication is the key to success. Legends like Winston Churchill, Abraham Lincoln and Martin Luther King made this their primary forte. More recently, Bill Clinton, Tony Blair, Narendra Modi and the founder of Isha Foundation, Jaggi Vasudev, (to name a few) have revelled in their communication prowess. Their skills were not only unmistakably effective with large audiences but in more private conversations as well. The question is: were they naturally endowed? Or did they consciously work on their abilities? Any natural ability needs further honing. It is a different matter that they may have worked with coaches who reoriented their styles, bit by bit. In the case of the ordinary man or woman, we are our own coaches by and large.

Unfortunately, not all of us change the way we communicate. Some get worse with the inclusion of harsh language, sarcasm and innuendos. These are people who never got useful feedback or who completely ignored it.

They could also be people who revel in contempt, sarcasm, showing someone in poor light, indignation or plain sadism. They are perhaps convinced that their usage of harsh language is equivalent to being no-nonsense and reckon it is non-malefic. What strange thinking! Perhaps their careers or family lives may not have been affected by what one would consider their 'uncultured' lexicon.

I salute the people who embrace positive changes in communication based on experiences and feedback. I was the perfect candidate for reshaping communication a few years ago. I knew one direct way of communicating, and that was it. I have changed it several times during my long career but have done so more decisively since entering Life 2.0. My move from accounting jobs to sales roles in my late twenties brought in the first round of changes. An accountant can afford to speak plainly, be brief and call a spade a spade. If anything, they must be more factual, sans emotions, and are paid to be that way. The English language gives us plenty of scope to spruce up our sentences to convey similar meanings with a less undesirable impact. As a salesperson in regular contact with team members and customers, social niceties are imbibed automatically. Facts are couched in gentler words, without casting aspersions on people or the system. If a customer cancelled an appointment, I used to apologize and remark that I shouldn't have rushed him into it, if it hadn't been the best day. As an accountant, however, I would have chastised a person who had cancelled the appointment for his poor professionalism. So, when the role changes, so does the behaviour.

My communication started getting better when I began dealing with some groups I had not dealt with before, such as students, fellow professors, business partners, board colleagues, school teachers, young children, etc. My exposure to these groups began in 2006 (when my Life 2.0 began). Each of these groups requires some sensitivity, poise, care, persuasion and emotive ingredients that I had to quickly integrate into my natural style. Try engaging a kindergarten child in a conversation for three minutes, without being authoritative! Try to patiently listen to your business partner who is senior to you, without interrupting him. Try to engage in a healthy give and take with fellow professors, especially when they have opposing views than yours. I had to learn all these with no teacher to teach and no time to waste. I am glad I shifted gears quickly and sought this higher order sensitivity, although it is still a work in progress. This conundrum is magnified, as there is no clear metric to assess the quality of communication. You need to assess it intuitively based on your personal yardstick or by keenly observing others who have mastered the skill.

Strategies that facilitate change

The following four strategies to facilitate change work for a lot of people, including me:

THE MANDATES: COORDINATES OF A NEW JOURNEY

- Deliberately using nice words, even if they may be simple ones like please, thank you, I appreciate..., etc. For example, a professor who I worked with would always start his feedback to a student's thesis presentation with the words, 'That was an excellent presentation.'
- Using questions instead of statements. For example, say 'Would you rather do it this way?' instead of saying 'Do it this way,' or even 'I prefer it that way.'
- Paraphrasing what has been heard and seeking confirmation at every stage. This is vital to ensure that the receiver's bias does not intrude into the conversation.
- Listening more than talking, in addition to listening better.

Listening well has enormous advantages that are often not even fully recognized. These have been enumerated below:

- You speak less and, by consequence, you speak less 'muck'.
- You can pick the language of the speaker to respond to him or her.
- You get valuable time to compose your responses, clearly and elegantly.
- You may find the speaker responding to many things himself or herself and you can choose what you need to respond to.
- You respect the speaker, which takes away much of the sting in the conversation.

- You do not expose your emotional weaknesses or impulses.
- You do not idle, the conversation still progresses.
- You empty your conversation partner.
- You gather a lot of data, which may be useful during the conversation or even later.
- You transfer the responsibility of maintaining a speaking etiquette on the other person.
- You get an opportunity to size up the other person, which is often important in negotiation, conflict resolution, etc.
- You get the opportunity to observe the partner's body language.
- The main tone of the conversation is set by the other person (lest you make a mistake by talking).
- It is considered the highest form of respect to the speaker.
- You understand better (plain and simple, isn't it?).

People consider listening as poor participation in a conversation and reckon that when they don't speak, they are not moving the conversation forward or not showing their control over the conversation. Nothing could be further from the reality. Our listening skill is often hampered in childhood, as eager parents want their children to speak early, speak more, speak smart and win arguments, all at the cost of not listening enough or carefully. So, when we try to improve, we are trying to eliminate a childhood habit, and that is often tough. Schools have exercises in listening comprehension to help form better listening habits and to help recall the text that has been listened to. Unfortunately, this dies down after early grades and is never encouraged further. There are no listening competitions, only speaking ones!

I am still not as good a listener as I would want to be, but the needle is moving. I am happier now that I have covered more ground than before. Watching other role models, the behaviour of people who tend to be quiet in a group, not watching the television cacophony or contrived conversations are some of the secrets to making progress on this front. Like everything else, you need to challenge yourself and want to change. People are quick to notice such a change and would compliment you if it is in the right direction. It also helps if you receive solicited or unsolicited feedback that you are prepared to accept. My daughter coached me in some ways to avoid what she called 'mansplaining'—the explanation of something by a man, typically to a woman, in a manner regarded as condescending or patronizing. In such a situation, we are at fault, even if our intention is good! It is similar to men giving driving directions (while the spouse is working it out her way) or men offering unsolicited advice on parking (reverse parking, especially). I have done them all myself and been told off for doing it! Listening to and acting on feedback is perhaps the best mode of improving communication or correcting less endearing statements.

Questions (rhetorical or otherwise) are a good way to

relay your wishes or preferences while making it seem like the other person's 'wise choice'. Kindergarten teachers often ask little children, 'Would you like to first put away your materials before going out to play?' This is a less dictating approach to communication. A question has the power to make the other person think and own the decision, something everyone wants in a conversation.

The maturing of communication is also reflected in our choice of the modes of communication. Many of us, as youngsters, treat a personal conversation and an email exchange as nearly equal, especially in professional settings. However, we gradually realize that there are very different outcomes to these modes. Depending on the situation, its sensitivity and the desired outcomes, it dawns on us later in life that emails can be dispensed with in many cases. My conversations with colleagues in the same campus is now 80 per cent personal, which means less misunderstandings, stonewalling, back-and-forth and acrimony, and faster resolution of issues.

Dale Carnegie very aptly said, 'There are always three speeches, for every one you actually gave. The one you practiced, the one you gave, and the one you wish you gave.' You can even add one more to these: 'The one you thought you gave.' Mature communication is a refreshing change for both the speaker and the audience (listener). In fact, when you reach that stage, you will wonder why people are less subtle and more offensive while communicating. Once again, Life 2.0 is a great point of time to recognize the issue and make this transition, although it could take some time to reach the ideal destination.

Good writing matters too

I have seen more pronounced changes in my written communication in Life 2.0. Miraculously, I developed an interest in writing. I write on and off for *The Business Times* in Singapore, and my first business book was published in 2018, followed by a self-improvement book in 2021. Writing is both a hobby and therapy for me. Most of my free time is devoted to three things: reading, writing or listening to Carnatic (South Indian classical) or film music. Writing is also a good surrogate for reflective thinking—this is a prerequisite for writing. Writing helps improve our language and hone our arguments and viewpoints, without having to be aggressive or bigoted. I have also utilized the opportunity to write to expand my interest into economics, geopolitics, policymaking, the digital world, etc. Readers are invisible (except when they comment), and hence, it is important to make a good guess of the readers' profiles, their likely interests, and match your language styles to theirs. For a couple of years, I read many issues of *The Financial Times*, *The New York Times* and *The Wall Street Journal* to understand the spectrum of writing styles, structures, tones, language simplicity, articulation and style of narration. I still read them when I travel. More than developing a style, I am happy about learning to connect the dots, form opinions, present them coherently (and with evidence) and draw appropriate insights and conclusions. I am sure this is considered elementary for writers (and for academic researchers). My joy comes from reaching that elementary stage of my own free will and with self-training. This process has also forced me to think of alternative phrases that are more objective and less judgmental. For example, if a colleague has not helped you enough in a project, while it is easy to say, 'You have not been helpful enough,' it is better to say, 'I might have gotten a better result with some more help from you.' There are even more polished (and gracious) versions like, 'I missed having your help and I am sure some circumstances must have come in your way.' When you put it this way, you are giving the person the benefit of doubt—what if the colleague had an unforeseen family event or an emergency at that time that kept him away from contributing? As written communication (even spoken, for that matter) cannot be erased, it is even more crucial to find the right balance between conveying a message and not offending the recipient. The mandates from the previous section on being grateful and gracious cannot be overemphasized in this context—being polite is a virtuous continuum.

Writing with a positive or neutral tone is easier than speaking that way, as you can review what you write before it is read by the recipient. I encourage my colleagues to compose their email, sleep on it, take another look, revise and then send the mail. This way, you can mitigate at least

50 per cent of any negative or unhappy responses.

The most testing times are when your communication is expected to be gracious but the circumstances are not otherwise friendly. Think of a scenario when you need to fire an employee. Writer Amanda Woodard suggests, 'Explain how you arrived at your decision, and infuse the whole thing with kindness by letting them know that you're sincerely sorry it hasn't worked out.'[44] You may think you don't need to, but given the unfavourable outcome for the other person, you have to walk the high ground. You gain a lot of credibility and understanding but lose nothing. Such sincere communication ensures that bridges are not burnt with the other person. Who knows? Perhaps you may cross paths again sometime somewhere!

Why do we need to embrace an evolved style of communication?

> *Half the world is composed of people who have something to say and can't, and the other half, who have nothing to say and keep on saying it.*
>
> —Robert Frost

Here are some reasons for us to embrace an evolved style of communication:

---

[44] Woodard, Amanda. 'In the firing line: How to dismiss an employee'. HRM. 2 March 2016. https://tinyurl.com/mv8ra3sn. Accessed on 4 April 2022.

- It helps us do our job better in a number of invisible ways.
- It strengthens our social relationships (for more on this, please read the ensuing section on social assets, page 140).
- It helps us reflect on how our performance as a communicator mirrors our character—whether we are nasty or uncivil.
- It gives us the ability to develop new skills like persuasion, conflict resolution, listening, graceful acceptance, objectivity, etc.
- It conditions our minds to new ways of looking at things. That is what books do as well.
- It provides a positive platform to engage new friends or new colleagues.
- It can be a good hobby. A good speaker charges fees up to a few thousand dollars per hour, and so do writers, counsellors, interlocutors, etc. These are all independent professions.
- It has the ability to enhance our likeability (do we ever think about it?).
- At the end of a long day of conversations or emails (if we escape unscathed from poor communication), it can be highly satisfying and is likely to leave us with less regrets.
- It is often the power source for mature handling of tough and delicate human situations and conflicts.
- It helps you keep up a virtuous learning cycle, which

- includes words, styles, tactics, behaviours, etc.
- It reflects our character and how we are judged (as Mark Twain puts it). I am sure we are keen on projecting the right image of ourselves.
- It may even advance our careers, just on its own merit! Communication is often the one thing that separates winners from losers.

It's not that we needed this volley of justifications to change our communication. We must have always felt our inadequacy or need for improvement. It is merely another nudge to take some concerted action to move forward. Perhaps it is time to do a reality check. Ask your peers and superiors at work or your family members at home how they would rate your communication on a scale of 1 to 10. Also ask them about what situations you excel at in communication and what situations bring out the devil in you. Write these down carefully, as they form your baseline before you initiate changes. The other starting point could be your own reflection of your past six months or one year to register how often you were misunderstood, how many times you had to argue, how frequently you alienated someone, how many times you came across as undignified and how many times your relationships had fissures! I hope your list does not go beyond a page! In this list, lie your low-hanging fruit to work towards.

For some, communication is the most essential factor for succeeding in their roles (professional or otherwise). Coaching people to excel in communication is now a paid profession, with step-by-step guidance being given to those who have asked to be helped. However, old habits don't leave us easily. Thus, we need a concerted action plan, with appropriate incentives and disincentives (to check for reversal). As we refine our communication, thereby increasing our likeability scores and perhaps even success in our endeavours, it sows the seed for a better legacy. Good communicators are remembered for it, and this is particularly true for corporate and political leaders.

Charity begins at home. Better communication at home is cheaper and easier to achieve—the people know you well and allow for trials and errors. It can become a practice ground, before you launch changes in the professional and external contexts. The more remarkable outcomes, however, come from professional and external contexts that move beyond your home because they reach many people. As with all the other mandates in the book, take conscious steps—today!

Working without Rewards

The highest reward for a person's toil is not what they get for it, but what they become by it.

—John Ruskin

'Becoming someone' is a central concept in legacy-making. Note that it differs a lot from other ideas like doing something or achieving something. In the latter ideas, the effect of the work on others and the society is not an automatic link. But working without rewards hands us that gift.

Rewards become an integral part of our lives from a very young age. We respond to tangible carrots better. The childhood candy, the teenage bicycle and the first car or overseas vacation in adulthood all belong to the same mould, something that extends to work life. When we are young working adults, financial rewards are strong motivators to do anything. Depending on our life and family circumstances, we are keen to upgrade ourselves and provide for ourselves and our immediate families. We pursue upward mobility in terms of comforts, symbols and indulgences. There is a popular reference to the goals of youngsters in Singapore (where I currently live)—the 5 Cs that refer to cash, car, credit card, condominium apartment and country club membership. All of these are money-driven comforts, and it's not surprising that young people are often motivated by these pursuits. Anything pro bono is less attractive during such a period, but it changes at some point. In some ways, a human being seldom acknowledges that he or she has reached financial immunity, which reduces the desire to seek a financial reward for everything. Yet, similar to delinking of finances and life, there comes a moment when you would like to take up some activities without expecting a quid pro quo—financial or otherwise. It could take simple forms like coaching the neighbour's kid in Mathematics or English, running errands for an ageing neighbour, doing some Sunday chores at a temple or church, helping traffic or crowd management at a major community event, etc. It could also lead to volunteering activities like collecting used clothing for orphanages, feeding the poor or spending time with senior citizens living in homes or living alone. At a further level, people indulge in business consulting for free, serving in committees that undertake community-centred art, music or drama programmes, practise law or medicine to support the underprivileged or for public causes, etc. Most of us are good citizens and are kindled by this thought, while only some put it to practice.

My mother, now 86, teaches classical music in the US to a few students as part of a temple's activities. She has forgone her salary as her donation to the temple activities, while the students pay fees to the temple. Her cumulative forgone salary over the past decade would exceed five figures in US dollars. This is her greatest source of satisfaction in her twilight years.

Activities like these have a few essential aspects—there is no vested interest (you are not doing it for a direct or indirect benefit), there is some quantifiable effort in terms of time, along with maybe money, and the activity is repetitive, usually not one-off. At one of the local Hindu temples that I visit, there is one soul who is a permanent volunteer. Natarajan (perhaps about 40) has a day job, but after 5.30 p.m., he is at the temple almost on all days, helping with the daily routines or supervising some activities during major events. His presence is conspicuous, but his manners are not. He is unassuming and has taken this activity up as an earnest form of prayer. To the best of my knowledge, he holds no official position at the temple nor does he work as a part of the temple team. He is the quintessential character that many Indian mythologies have—a benefactor without an identity. Film music genius, A. R. Rahman, in his Oscar acceptance speech, said, 'All glory and fame is to God.'[45] The spiritual guidebook, Bhagavad Gita, talks about doing one's duty without expecting anything in return (or forgoing the returns to God). Natarajan is a good follower of this principle. Last year, he was seen as active as ever, with a sling around his fractured arm. The motivation to do this 365 days a year must be a strong inner call. If you don't believe in its challenge, try doing this for 10 consecutive days!

The impetus to undertake such activities can be triggered at any age. The seeds for such activities are sown in the mind early, but people tend to ideate such tasks in their minds and postpone action till one of the following occurs:

- A good friend goads you into doing something that your mind is already set on.
- A sudden freeing up of your time presents an opportunity.
- A hurdle is removed (time slot or commuting difficulties, for example).
- A pilot opportunity comes up (to try first before committing to an opportunity).

---

[45] Press Trust of India. 'Rahman dedicates Oscars to god, mother', *The Times of India*, 23 February 2009, https://tinyurl.com/482bkhn9. Accessed on 4 April 2022.

- Other life interests suddenly (or gradually) do not seem to be fulfilling.
- You get inspired by a guru (increasingly).
- It's a calling of sorts. If you are processing it in your mind, it means you are ready for it.

Irrespective of these, the proverbial question remains: how and when do you act?

Life 2.0 was the point at which my mind wandered towards such a purpose. It was the confluence of delinking finances and life, freeing up of time (now that I was away from a hectic corporate career) and a desire to do something without a reward while I am still fully able. Three activities excited me—coaching youngsters, organizing music events and writing. I am involved in all of these in some ways now. In the beginning, I signed up to teach English to an underprivileged family (with three young kids) whose parents were uneducated. I could only do it for about 18 months, as scheduling issues curtailed the continuity. But the experience was motivating and humbling. The family could not afford private tuition nor could the children manage to have a decent collection of books. I had to learn to engage curious but playful kids between the ages of four and eight in serious activities like reading, without making them monotonous. I was getting better at those skills when it tapered off during a holiday break.

Along with a couple of other like-minded friends, I helped open a new organization that conducted chamber and public concerts of Carnatic music in Singapore. The organization has completed its tenth year and has held four major festivals, where top artists have performed. Even though a large amount of preparatory and event-centric work is done by a handful of people, it is absolutely a labour of love. The finances are always tight (sometimes balanced with contributions from promoters), but the quality has been kept high. Most of the paid public events attract a crowd of over 500 listeners. I have retreated to an advisory role in the past couple of years, as some young Turks have come in to manage the logistics and operations very skilfully. I helped the organization host about three to four chamber events per year, most of which were held at my home. We added themes to the events and cast our net wide to include a number of good local artists. We incurred some expenses too, and it, therefore, involved working without rewards! We have now successfully extended this festival to virtual concerts due to the crowd restrictions during the pandemic.

Some of my writing is pro bono or comes with miniscule remuneration. However, it is a time-consuming activity. I have expanded my interests to include music criticism, economics, the digital world, etc. My critiques of music concerts cost me more in terms of commuting and time than my token compensation for such pieces. However, that income has never been the motive. When you take up such activities, you would notice that it may entail going beyond a pastime into a commitment. I am also involved in a significant funding and advisory activity for an important social cause in India, which I don't discuss generally. I think

I have only scratched the surface of this idea, which has enormous happiness and satisfaction potential. I am thankful for these opportunities and for the desire to take them up. I chose pursuits that fit my interests and competencies. That's not unusual and I am sure many readers have embraced such pursuits without a whisper.

It is also not uncommon for working pro bono to be institutionalized. At Arnold & Porter, one of the leading legal firms in the US, all lawyers have to do 15 per cent pro bono work.[46] That is a lot more than the 2 per cent corporate social responsibility (CSR) profit share that has been recently mandated in India.[47] Besides, the activity is expected to be performed at each individual's level. Top legal firms, their lawyers and partners earn handsome fees. This firm, however, likes to foster a culture of giving back to the society in the form of legal support to those in need. That such pro bono work is built into the work life is further advantageous since no special plan is needed to work without rewards.

One of the best examples of renouncing the reward of one's deeds is the legendary South Indian classical singer M.S. Subbulakshmi.[48] In a career spanning about 60 years,

---

[46] 'Pro Bono', Arnold & Porter, https://tinyurl.com/59h932m6. Accessed on 4 April 2022.

[47] ENS Economic Bureau. 'Mandatory 2% CSR spend set to kick in from April 1', *The Indian Express*, 28 February 2014, https://tinyurl.com/4uffmfvn. Accessed on 4 April 2022.

[48] 'MS Subbulakshmi—Giving generously of her music', Carnaticography, https://tinyurl.com/yu6dum25. Accessed on 4 April 2022.

THE MANDATES: COORDINATES OF A NEW JOURNEY 135

she won many awards and was well-remunerated for concerts, almost all of which were donated for causes like education, healthcare, poverty alleviation programmes, and other human and religious causes. There is no parallel to this anywhere in the world. Her legacy is, thus, a glorious amalgamation of divine music and selfless, compassionate deeds. Perhaps it's unthinkable to emulate such renunciation of rewards. That she lived a simple and often financially challenged existence makes it even more peerless. People like her are born once in a blue moon.

Working without rewards can sometimes shift your priorities significantly, in some cases, completely. During Life 2.0, this may even lead to a change of careers. People have moved from paying professions to non-paying community causes. Such examples are even more dramatic than others that we see regularly. The homemaker is often cited as an example of the greatest selfless worker who manages a myriad of chores at home, caring for all the family members for the non-monetary reward of her family's happiness!

When working without rewards, there is also a potential battle with our ego. When we engage in such work, do we always do it without publicity? Or is there a desire for being in the limelight and for society to shower us with appreciation? So, even if money is not the motive, something else is. With social media publicity being so freely available, the temptation to seek attention is strong. That does not fit in with the spirit of this mandate.

Chapter 3, verse 19 of the Bhagavad Gita highlights

the selfless nature of service through the concept of karma yoga, 'Therefore, giving up attachment, perform actions as a matter of duty because by working without being attached to the fruits, one attains the Supreme.'[49]

We need to draw a distinction between volunteering, which only involves donating money, and working, which involves our minds, bodies, time, intellectual capacity, skills, initiative, organizational ability, etc. The latter is harder, and I find that for every person who is willing to pledge to this, there are about a few hundred people who can just write cheques. As discussed in the section on impacting society, the real test of your attitude towards society, in my opinion, comes from non-monetary engagement. At the school that I cofounded, we organize projects for young students to spend their time and energy on such rewardless societal pursuits, sometimes on weekends. The world has generally more donors than doers. Ask Bill and Melinda Gates—they would tell you the difficulties of translating their generous grants into impactful and sustainable change in places like Africa. The social support activities on the ground are the ones that desperately need better managerial talent, strategies and concerted and passionate labour.

The Satya Sai organization at Puttaparti, Andhra Pradesh, and its other centres in India,[50] are another good

---

[49]'Bhagavad Gita: Chapter 3, Verse 19', Bhagavad Gita: The Song of God, https://tinyurl.com/ynn65d7p. Accessed on 4 April 2022.
[50]Sri Sathya Sai Central Trust, https://tinyurl.com/ynycdcza. Accessed on 4 April 2022.

example. Here, people sign up as volunteers for service and get assigned periodic duties at the centres to manage crowds at the prayer sessions or to participate in serving free food or other chores, all of which are efforts with no monetary reward or identity. The scale of the movement is breathtaking as is the discipline that is ingrained in its character. It continues undiminished long after the spiritual founder and guru has passed on. I have friends who have enrolled in this mission and do not want to be disturbed with any other activity (including family routines) on the days that they dedicate to the organization. They even rearrange travel schedules so that no appointment to serve is missed. For these volunteers, work and the opportunity to serve are the rewards. It's not a one-off engagement as many of the volunteers are long-term servants.

Benefits of working without rewards

There are a number of benefits to working without rewards, especially without the financial ones.

- Your life is not spent only caring about yourself and your immediate family. You contribute to the larger society. We discussed this in the section on impacting society (see page 23) as well, but the additional angle here is foregoing any reward.
- You are often a volunteer who does not hold any position of authority (unlike your primary career). That has a sobering effect on the ego and builds

people skills, as opposed to authority-based influence.
- You come to appreciate the privileges that you enjoy vis-à-vis the others you engage with, including the people who are yet to make their mark in their lives.
- Your involvement in these activities seems to actually increase your longing for such pursuits. You may begin to realize that financial rewards are not everything. The Natarajans of the world keep inspiring you.
- Your focus on yourself reduces dramatically since there is no time for self-indulgence, self-pity, self-promotion, attention craving, etc. The focus is outside you. This is a good state to be in, if you can sustain it.
- Your alternate skills are put to test. Can you do anything other than your regular job? Can you work with young children? Can you patiently spend hours with ageing people? Can you manage a large public gathering? Can you plan for an event with major financial uncertainty? Can you bring yourself to do blue-collar tasks? (See the section on learning new skills, page 4).
- Somehow the labour of love brings a paradoxical form of satisfaction that is different from your day job, for which you are actually remunerated. It could be attributed to a combination of working against the odds with new people in abstract and unfamiliar situations, seeing the way your work benefits others and witnessing the power of volunteerism.
- You have an outlet for your talents that may not be

monetizable. We all have plenty of such abilities.
- You can seek to become a role model for your children or family around you. Do discuss your engagement in such activities with children to sow the seeds of rewardless work in their minds too.
- The society starts to look at you differently and sees you as an inspiration.
- You are on your way to becoming an 'ideal' person.

These benefits are largely for the soul and lead to a better conscience. For many people, there comes the point of flux when life moves more and more towards such activities and away from typical paying careers. In actual practice, this begins as a parallel pursuit to your day job and has the potential to evolve into a full routine. In some cases, you can do both—earn while you work for others, which satisfies you to the same degree.

Child psychologists argue that linking children's activities to rewards (grades, certificates or other physical forms) robs them of the intrinsic motivation to learn and be competent. Experiments with an incentivized group and a non-incentivized group have underlined these theories. Thus, the psychological concept of 'operant conditioning',[51] which is often deployed to train animals, is discouraged for humans. If the trend of service without returns catches on truly, children could grow up to naturally embrace the

---

[51] 'Operant Conditioning (B.F. Skinner)', InstructionalDesign.org, https://tinyurl.com/3fh7ajs8. Accessed on 4 April 2022.

doctrine of working without rewards.

In the corporate world, young managers are often advised to take on additional roles without any additional rewards in order to progress to the top of the line for promotions and higher responsibilities. The initiative and sacrifices are never forgotten.

Those who have only heard about these stories of working without rewards must now begin to do the same, hopefully with conviction. Choose a neighbourhood support group and pledge a few Saturdays to its activities to the best of your abilities. Evaluate the experience, especially how you feel about it. It will be hard to stop you from continuing. Every person who benefits from your pro bono work will thank you in their hearts—that's a worthy legacy to aspire for.

Acquiring Social Assets

A classmate of mine from business school has a unique knack of building warm relationships with anyone around. While at school, he was a normal student from a humble background, and yet, he managed to win the contested post of student leader. All the votes were personally sought out and won. Fast forward 25 years, when our batch's silver jubilee reunion was announced, he took the initiative, reached out to several classmates in far-flung continents and managed to get 70 per cent of our batch (most of them with their spouses) to the campus for a two-day retreat! That was a record number in over 20 years of such reunions. My friend never really lost touch with our batchmates. When he travelled, he found batchmates in the town that he was visiting and asked them to meet him for a cup of coffee or a meal. He interviewed some of the more successful ones and featured them in the monthly alumni magazine. Unsurprisingly, he took charge of reporting our batch news. He has done this over the past three decades while looking after his own career and family, not to mention a PhD that he completed later in life. He did all of these in the pre-social-media era, with limited avenues for staying in touch.

His likeability factor did not come from his academic exploits, family background, magnetic personality or high-flying career. It was a combination of soft factors—his warmth, genuine friendship, constant outreach, concern and care. His joys and sorrows are always shared by the community of batchmates. This is the formidable degree to which he has built his social assets. In fact, he is often the first name anyone from my batch thinks of in Mumbai, his city of residence. True to his character, it should be said that he has not exploited any of the contacts for personal objectives. What is this phenomenon? What prompted him to take it up as a lifelong passion? If there was no pecuniary gain, what did he achieve with this grand network? The answers to these questions have to be carefully curated.

What is a social asset? It is a constructed web of social relationships—some intimate, some distant and many in between—that you create and nurture to varying degrees over a period of time. These relationships are called assets because they have the capacity to bring you returns! We will study this phenomenon in detail.

We are never complete without our friends. Unfortunately, the words 'friends', 'acquaintances' and 'casual introductions' have all been somewhat jumbled up in our minds. As words get thrown around, we even have 'best friends'! What would you call a person that you met once or twice and conversed with for a limited duration? Can you classify him or her as a friend? The social media terminologies have also polluted the real worth of 'links' and 'friends'. In this amorphous world of friends, social assets have become blurred. Worse still, such assets are measured in quantifiable metrics—likes, views, comments, etc. Does that measure our social capital? Certainly not. There has to be a deeper meaning to the relationship in order for it to be called a social asset. That is, a relationship that does not diminish significantly over a period of time and one which has mutuality of interest sustaining it. How many of your relationships (links included) will stand the test of mutuality?

We must first accept that one of the greatest meanings and purposes of life is sharing. We discussed sharing of knowledge and expertise earlier. What about sharing experiences, happiness, moods, feelings, sources of joy, enlightenment and companionship? On the face of it, they have no material value to us. Yet, when we reflect on it, we will realize that mankind keeps reminding us about this glorious opportunity to be in a social construct, which we ignore and spurn all the time but for a few. When all other assets have been acquired, we may find that we do not have many people to share our joys with. This cruel truth strikes many of us rather late!

Learning from other species and creations

Nature teaches us the perfect lesson. California is famous for the iconic redwood forests that are often referred in superlatives—they are the tallest, highest, oldest, most connected, etc. The trees are over 100 metres tall, with a girth of perhaps 3 metres. Some have stood in this forest for over 3,000 years and have weathered many natural calamities like winds, storms, earthquakes, etc. Yet, most of them have survived. They are not necessarily the most deep-rooted trees though. What is the secret of their growth and longevity? They are together. Yes, their shallow roots spread around and intertwine with those of their neighbours and form an interconnected network that gives them the combined strength to be durable and big.[52] They secure their future by being together.

All natural things around us are connected—the meadows, the trees, the earth, the animals that walk on them, the flowers, water, air, sunlight, darkness in the night, birds and insects, and all living and non-living things. There seems to be a perfect ecosystem where each one of these

---

[52] 'About Coast Redwoods', California Department of Parks and Recreation, https://tinyurl.com/2p8r4j8e. Accessed on 4 April 2022.

creatures and elements interact with each other in their own way and exist collectively. This is so imbibed in their nature that it has now become a pattern that is millions of years old. Their connections are smooth, mutual and unconditional. Many of the animals and birds, in fact, move in tandem, eat together and share habitats. Collectivism is an asset for them. However, that can't be said of human beings. More often than not, we are keen to disconnect than connect.

Why should social assets be built at all? Apart from our affiliation needs that are mentioned in Abraham Maslow's hierarchy, there is a great potential for us to earn legacy points with a strong social capital. Many social assets may become your well-wishers, fans, mentors, mentees, caregivers, walking or conversational companions, and so on. With the consolidation of such a relationship and sharing of experiences and anecdotes, your life story is preserved for posterity in the minds of those who outlive you. Even if everyone is not a plot point for your biography, writers turn to intimate friends for information on the person they seek to portray. The social capital we build is also a possible fountain of opportunities for us that may lead to other mandates in this book, like coaching, impacting society, learning new skills, reshaping communication, etc. We learn from our buddies and learn better by observing and modelling others. Just like the unique person that we are, so is our social asset base!

As I mentioned earlier, there is a strong connection between the mandates in this book. For example, it was proved in a paper published by the National Center for Biotechnology Information (NCBI),[53] a part of the National Institute of Health in the US, that expressing gratitude to a new person increases the chances of that person seeking a sustained relationship with you. Therefore, it should be quite easy to say thanks to a few people every week and open the doors to social asset-building. Some medical professionals believe in the therapeutic effect of intimate friends on the recovery of ailing people.

Not the same as transactional contacts

One always hears that some people consider themselves well-networked. The nature of such networks needs to be understood. Is this network largely fashioned out of professional needs (on both sides) or does it not have a quid pro quo? Is there a natural appeal towards each other or is it forced by circumstances or transactional interests? It is possible that in Life 1.0, we may have gravitated towards relationships that are linked to our professions and transactional interests (a good colleague, a lawyer friend, a banker contact, a local government official, a financial advisor, a family physician, etc.). This is not uncommon. Some of these relationships may qualify to become the social

---

[53] Williams, Lisa A., Bartlett, Monica Y. 'Warm thanks: gratitude expression facilitates social affiliation in new relationships via perceived warmth', *Emotion*, Vol. 15, No. 1, 2015, 1-5. https://tinyurl.com/2p998fdn. Accessed on 4 April 2022.

asset that we are referring to here. In the fast-moving first-half of life, we may ignore the long-term needs of social capital, even as many of the transactional acquaintances disappear from our circle. Our interest here, therefore, is to discuss 'true' social assets.

So, how do we know where we stand on this mandate? Try this exercise: list all your achievements over the years (you will know which ones to consider and which ones to leave out). It could be academic honours, workplace commendations, extracurricular pursuits, spouse introductions, public honours, recovery from an uncertain phase or tragedy, financial successes, personal milestones, family successes, other laurels and even dangers that you have avoided. Those that altered the course of your life or career may be the first ones you think of, but there may be other less striking events or moments as well. Alongside each, write the names of people who may have played some part in your success or recovery—family members, colleagues, mentors, strangers, childhood friends, teachers, bosses, adversaries, etc. If your list is not long, I bet you haven't thought hard or are unwilling to acknowledge the roles played by others in what you reckon are your achievements. Even if their contributions are not major, they would have mattered. Such individuals may have played a role in introductions, recommendations, mentoring, advisory or other forms of support. I am not suggesting that only if you got something out of someone, he or she qualifies to be an asset. That merely confirms the quality of the relationship.

Your social assets and their relative character should be evident from such a list. Many of these people would have crossed paths with you somewhat haphazardly and without any real planning. Life 2.0 is a turning point to seek and accumulate more social assets. This requires some soul-searching into how we have managed our relationships so far. There is a small minority that does this exceptionally well even in Life 1.0—we can learn a lot from them. Relationship experts categorize most relationships into the following categories:

- strongly sustained over a long period of time (there is a tinge of permanence to such relationships);
- has seen better days and has waned or even vanished (such relationships are spoken of in the past tense);
- undergoes frequent volatility and never settles down but never ends either;
- is in a developmental phase and needs extensive tender, love and care to grow;
- was once very strong but died inexplicably (or due to a clash);
- continues at a steady pace with no strong nurturing inputs (a naturalized bond);
- is called upon once in a while but remains in the loop despite no regular contact.

Draw a pie chart of all your relationships to see how they are distributed across these seven categories. You are doing very well, if 1, 6 and 7 are the dominant categories. There is an inherent strength if these dominate. We are looking for quality, resilience and strength rather than just numbers. You need more analysis, reflection and resetting, if the others are dominant. You may have heard about relationships that fall into categories 1, 2 or 3 as network contacts in the professional context. The social asset categorization for such relationships is vastly different and nuanced.

Reasons for a weak social assets base

If you think seriously about the underlying factors behind why your pie chart does not reflect strong social assets, you will understand that:

- You are not consciously building up this asset.
- You take a transactional approach rather than a relationship approach to the people in your circle (for more details, see page 150).
- You try to maintain too many relationships simultaneously. Thus, you are not able to do justice to building or growing the asset qualitatively.
- You neglect relationships that need a booster shot.
- You do not balance the mutuality of interests (perhaps you are more interested and the other person is not).
- You do not sort out any misunderstanding early enough.
- You constantly drift away to newer connections (this is a natural phenomenon, as our friend circles change with time, place and profession).

- You have destroyed the edifice of your relationships by seeking too many favours. While favours and help are part of any equation, there is always a limit that can lead to a breakdown, if breached.
- You may cause some damage by seeking dominance in the relationship.
- You may unwittingly (or wittingly) trample the oath of secrecy that is associated with social assets.
- You do not stick to your end of the bargain (contacts, co-activities, etc.). Ever postponed a lunch with a friend half a dozen times?
- You feel competitive pressures in relationships (seeing win–lose pictures).
- You trade your social asset for your ego.
- You are caught in the crossfire of a rivalry between a family member and a friend's family member (rivalries among children or spouses are more common).
- You may be reclusive and not realize the loss of social assets (only those who give up normal life do this intentionally).
- You are so obsessed with other goals that you have lost sight of this goal or it has slipped to the periphery of your goals.
- You develop a competitive rivalry (real or imagined).
- You receive wisdom that discourages social relationships.

With so many potential causes for failures and missteps, it is natural that the social asset graph is never going to be smooth or on a positive trajectory. So, do we want to fix that? Could we consider the point of Life 2.0 to address it more deliberately?

My list of who I would call social assets consist of about 60–70 people (which surely sounds limited), if I exclude some immediate family members who would certainly qualify for it. I probably would have about 30–35 people who could be categorized in categories 1, 6 and 7 mentioned earlier. I am unable to create a benchmark for myself, but I have reached the unsurprising conclusion that I hold fewer assets than most people. I am currently introspecting on how I could have done better. I have initiated a few things, thanks to connectivity options like LinkedIn and WhatsApp to seek out some old friends, meet my classmates whenever I visit their towns, proactively offer to share interesting material (that I know they may like), pick up the phone and call people I haven't spoken to for decades, introspect on dormant or waning relationships, etc. I have come to realize that building social assets needs concerted and focused efforts, and changes to one's communication preferences. I now try to reply to almost all the emails from friends, even if some come with requests that I may not be able to fulfil. Similarly, I am starting to reach out to people I may have neglected in the past. I am nudging myself to forgive old misunderstandings and seek new beginnings with some people. I feel good about the changes I am making to achieve a better social asset pool. I hope to have some good results in two to three years.

THE MANDATES: COORDINATES OF A NEW JOURNEY 151

One of the problems of Life 1.0 is the singular focus on positive outcomes for us or for our immediate families in everything we do. This often results in a transactional approach with the people we meet. Everyone is perceived to have a utility value for us and the direction and magnitude of relationship is directly proportional to the perception of their utility. When their utility diminishes, so does the value of the social asset to us. For example, you and your young family may have moved cities (or even countries) and met some people who formed the initial support system for you. They advise you about where to live, who is a good family physician, which schools to look at and even find a nanny for your little one. They may drive you around to settle several things for you and initiate you into social circles that you may like. A couple of years later, you hardly meet them or keep in touch until you hear that an elderly person from the family, who you had met occasionally, has passed away. How do you feel at that point? It sounds like an opportunistic engagement in a way and may be relatable to many readers.

In his bestselling book, Reid Hoffman, the co-founder of LinkedIn, talks about the effect of having strong and weak ties.[54] He and his co-author introduce the concept of 'network literacy', an acquired skill of expanding your connections. He also elaborates on the idea of doing someone a favour in order to earn that person's friendship. In reality, we seldom do that because our prism is fitted with

---

[54] The Start-Up of You, https://tinyurl.com/2d34zaf2. Accessed on 4 April 2022.

glass panes that do not reflect the outside view. Therefore, we let go of several opportunities to expand our social capital. The more interesting part of the book is about how our less intense community of friends also represent capital that is useful in ways that we cannot even imagine.

As another exercise, draw up a list of people who were reasonably 'close' to you in the past but have drifted away, mostly because you have nothing to 'gain' from the association anymore. That number will shake you out of your slumber. Through this exercise, you may infer that your social assets have, in fact, been depleting, mostly due to a transactional approach, neglect and changes to your needs.

My late grandparents have been wonderful role models for me in this aspect. They came from lower-middle-class backgrounds and took it upon themselves to help and support others who were in need. My grandfather ran a virtual pro bono employment bureau and would recommend many 18-year-old boys in search of employment for jobs in Mumbai in the fifties and sixties. In their 500 sq. ft. apartment, many people would stay for short periods, before they attained economic stability. My grandmother would throw a hearty feast (all with her own labour and limited means) for any friend visiting the city. Their mission to be helpful to others was legendary. Their social asset base was wider than that of anyone that I have known. They built it with their own efforts, not from any privileged position or a legacy. It was almost their only goal in life, and as it turned out, their only asset! In their sunset days, almost everyone would visit them frequently, thanks to their warmth and hospitality. This happened despite it being the era of less connectivity. My grandparents assumed that this was the simplest help they could offer with least impact on their wallets. Little did they realize that they had built up a huge social edifice. I am not sure how you would quantify that return of capital. They have both passed away, but the next generation is enjoying the same connections to some degree. When my family and friends celebrated my grandfather's centenary (long after he had passed on), more than 500 people turned up. That's the perfect legacy many would cherish.

Here is a morbid but pertinent thought. One of the secret wishes of most people is being well eulogized by people around them and by as many people as possible. It is verily the declaration of your legacy. So, what will fetch you such a legacy? This is usually the harvest of the social assets that you sow. We take nothing material from this world, we only take with us fond recollections, praises, memories of time spent together and encomiums of others about us.

Irving Berlin, one of America's greatest songwriter-composers, wrote, 'The song is ended but the melody lingers on...' This melody is the reverberation of your social assets. So, how does one build (or rebuild) the 'ideal' social asset base? There are plenty of books and advice on this subject. One of the key principles is that you should be likeable. It may be a strange thought, but I have seen some people who go out of their way to make themselves difficult to like. I am also convinced about one other thing. Even though relationships can't be viewed as a quid pro quo, in actual practice, what goes around does come around. When you help, support, inspire or invest in some people and activities, you somehow redeem it in different forms from others who may be completely unconnected. This need not be just help in return, but companionship, counsel and a support ecosystem in another phase of life. It is akin to the karma principle, but returned within the same life. In fact, there is a Tamil proverb that translates to, 'What you do in the morning can be harvested in the afternoon,' and this applies to both good and bad deeds.

We also lose a lot of capital over time. 'So yes, I have lost some good friends, and this is what hurts me the most,'[55] says Dr Sudha Murthy, chairperson of Infosys Foundation, a prolific author and philanthropist. She refers to her changed wealth status (courtesy her billionaire husband, Mr Narayana Murthy, co-founder of Infosys) as a possible factor. As relationships sour or become less important or as our relative social positions change, we drift away from people. Can you restore a soured relationship? This is linked to a later section on moderating the ego (see page 166). In some ways, re-establishing a previous relationship is easier than building a new one. This is similar to the merits of serving an existing customer better rather than acquiring a new customer (a B2B maxim).

---

[55]Press Trust of India. 'Sudha Murthy: A tale of less old friends and no new saree!', *Business Standard*, 30 July 2017, https://tinyurl.com/4wxw28bt. Accessed on 4 April 2022.

Paradoxically, the COVID-19 pandemic brought people closer together in spirit, even though physical distancing was the norm. Most of us found enough time and enthusiasm to revisit old friends and caught up virtually with them. Our common interests and passions were reignited (music, art, stories, etc.), and it brought people closer. I now have subgroups within my bigger WhatsApp groups, whose members have some common interests, which develop a deeper degree of closeness.

The feel-good effect of building one's social assets is indescribable. New people bring new perspectives, rules, languages, feelings and anchors. You are constantly learning to enhance your relationship skills. It does take a toll on time and other priorities. But nothing comes without focused effort, and that remains the essence of this book.

In some ways, social assets can be built by just correcting our omissions and commissions rather than undertaking a mammoth new effort that some of the other mandates need. In that sense, building social assets has the quickest payback and most visibility.

Being Ourselves

> *All the world's a stage, and all the men and women merely players.*
>
> —William Shakespeare, Act 2, Scene 7,
> *As You Like It*

We are all actors on the large stage of mankind. Each of us takes a form, assumes a role, which brings with it the norms of how that role must be played. The problem is that most times, we add our own wishes and desires to that role. One such desire is to be seen as 'someone' by others. However, that 'someone' may or may not be our true self. We encounter this situation all through our lives.

A school student may try to pass off as affluent when, in fact, he or she is not. The motivation to do such a thing is to be included in certain circles. A college student may subscribe to a certain social view, even if privately he or she does not agree with it. This time the motivation may be not being excluded from mainstream groups or to be part of the popular discourse. This pattern continues at every stage in life—adulthood, family, job, etc. We may or may not be aware of our level of pretension because it starts to become a habit. It is a projection of what you are not or what you do not subscribe to.

Wearing this mask reflects several cravings that we may have, including seeking approval for ourselves or our actions, blending in without attracting undue attention, wanting to appear perfect (physically and metaphorically), creating an unnaturally perfect social media profile to gain favourable attention, etc. We may justify it as peer pressure and an essential part of the social scheme. These justifications give us sweeping legitimacy for 'acting' in real life. The 'acting life' is, thus, a parasite that can go beyond limits and slowly erode our original character.

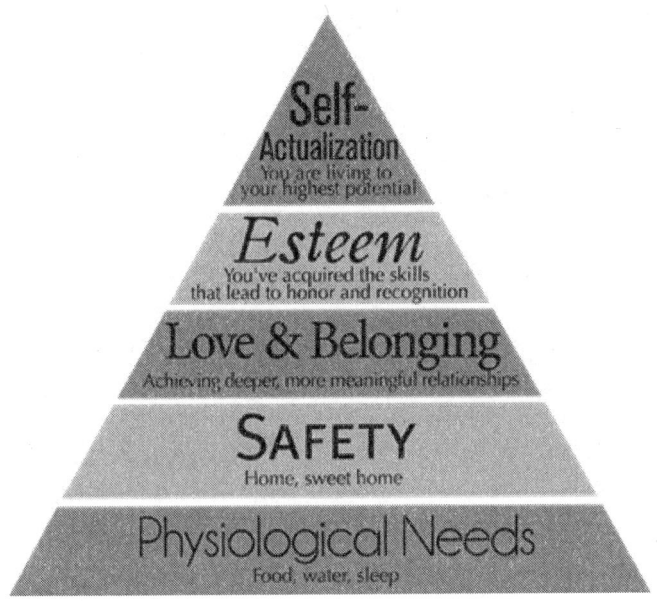

Maslow's hierarchy of needs
Source: Education Library[56]

In the pyramid of Abraham Maslow's hierarchy of human needs, social needs come ahead of self-esteem or self-actualization needs. Our actions are a product of these social needs. Is there an escape from this? What are the long-term implications of non-stop acting?

A stag, drinking from a crystal spring, saw his reflection in the clear water. He greatly admired the graceful arch of

---

[56]Kurt, Serhat. 'Maslow's Hierarchy of Needs in Education', *Education Library*, 6 February 2020, https://tinyurl.com/2p9fyuff. Accessed on 4 April 2022.

his antlers, but he was ashamed of his spindling legs. 'How can it be,' he sighed, 'that I should be cursed with such legs when I have so magnificent a crown.' At that moment, he caught the scent of a panther, and in an instant, was bounding away through the forest. However, as he ran, his wide-spreading antlers got caught in the branches of the trees, and soon the panther overtook him. Then, the stag observed that the legs that he was so ashamed of would have saved him had it not been for the useless ornaments on his head.

A quote from the Aesop's fables sums this up aptly, 'We often make much of the ornamental and despise the useful.'[57] This is a symbolic story of how we seek another version of ourselves rather than the original. Besides the inner conflict that it invites, this behaviour has a debilitating influence on how our unique persona manifests (or not).

Does the need for status trigger pretension?

An important attribute of success is to be yourself. Never hide what makes you, you.

—Indra Nooyi, former Chairperson and CEO, PepsiCo

Some people (I reckon it is more common in Asian societies) go to great lengths to portray a persona of themselves that

---

[57]'The Stag at the Pool', *Fables of Aesop,* https://tinyurl.com/stag-at-the-pool. Accessed on 4 April 2022.

is artificially contrived. The excuse is to convey a status and the acts are symbols of that explanation. Mercedes Benz and BMW sell more cars in China than their home country, Germany. The car you drive, the home you own (especially the location), the schools your children go to, the watch you wear, the brand of suit you wear, your holiday destinations, the pen that you use to sign documents are all such symbols. This is, in fact, the idea behind marketing luxury goods to those who are not necessarily rich—they are wannabes! Many would say that there isn't anything wrong with that idea. Not at all! It is, after all, a personal choice. The point is whether it is the norm or a periodic (or regular) aberration for an individual.

Thus, the key question is: are you pretending so much that your real persona is largely hidden? Are you trapped in a situation that conditions your mind to think of external optics every time? If you are, you can't resist the temptation to continue doing it. There is, sometimes, a skewed argument that such acting pays off because it helps us progress professionally or financially.

We need to be original and stand for our true selves. That's the resting place for our conscience. The drive to decorate our persona, if it is led by the desire for external recognition, will lead to a conflict of the conscience. It is not very different from the other choices we face in life—career, life partner, etc. In all these cases, do we not allow our natural wisdom and inclination to prevail?

Author, speaker and CEO, Peter Bregman, said, 'I now

care less what other people think and more about what things feel like to me. I'm calmer. Less needy of praise. I speak and act more deliberately. The immensity of the change has been startling to me'[58] Talking about leadership traits, it is often said that a leader who does not hide his weakness is actually strong, invites collaboration and trust and stays human. No one is perfect, and your team will understand that. It is also possible that the people around you actually know your weakness, even if you have never admitted it. Being yourself and acknowledging your frailties increase your acceptability and invite better cooperation.

The public persona and conflicts

> *If you compare yourself with others,*
> *you may become vain and bitter;*
> *for always there will be greater and lesser persons*
> *than yourself.*
> *Enjoy your achievements as well as your plans.*
>
> —Max Ehrmann[59]

Our public act is not without its conflicts. Should we be normative in a given social context or be ourselves (if that is

---

[58] Bregman, Peter. 'Who are you really mad at?', *Harvard Business Review*, 23 July 2012, https://tinyurl.com/4chjjf8v. Accessed on 4 April 2022.

[59] Ehrmann, Max. 'Desiderata-Words for Life', All Poetry, https://tinyurl.com/5n7ptvr6. Accessed on 4 April 2022.

different)? We may face this question in the context of dress codes (most of the world has moved to Western dress codes), public etiquettes, language subtleties, group behaviours, relationship rules, grace principles, etc. Practices in your town, country, neighbourhood, sub-class could largely govern your attitude to these aspects, and some conflict may be inevitable if you wish to insist on your natural instinct. In the larger context of our behaviour, these are minor things. They come and go, and don't necessarily inflict permanent alterations to our persona. It is, thus, possible to stay with the crowd on some things and be ourselves on most other substantive matters.

As Eleanor Roosevelt, former first lady of the United States, famously stated, 'No one can make you feel inferior without your consent.' How many of you can relate to this? I certainly can. The desire to come across as knowledgeable, the urge to impress, the craving for praise, the instinct to enhance the projection of outshining others, claiming wrongful credit, an exaggerated sense of self-importance are all elements of the grand action. I must admit that I have been swept away by such needs at some moments. Fortunately, by the time I realized it and started making some corrections, I had not gone too far. Luckily, it wasn't my default behaviour. It was an exception, but one that I had repeated many times over. To some extent, the correction came after reflecting on the outcomes of such behaviour, once its ego-massaging effect started feeling futile, and one accepted the consequences of being oneself. God has created over seven billion beautiful, unique entities. He didn't want us to be someone else, and why should we be?

Apple founder Steve Jobs has talked about how he had to get past naysayers and failures to uphold his self-belief in his ideas and actions. We know his story of steep falls and colossal rises. His not allowing his normal self to be cowed down is an example that fits into our argument very well. We don't stand up when we give up.

If the mask or the veneer is a substantive trait of an individual, it may potentially have some unpleasant consequences. A college student in the US took her life as she felt she had gone too far posing for others, and it became unsustainable for her, creating too much inner conflict. Plagiarism, cheating, robbery, etc., are some dire outcomes of trying to be someone else, and looking for quick or better outcomes than what our natural self can achieve. Scientists may fabricate favourable results of their experiments in order to claim honours that otherwise may not have been achievable. Academic papers founded on surveys have sometimes been challenged for bias and doctored findings. The motives behind breaching the principles of honesty are clearly linked to seeking fame desperately or being out of sync with our abilities.

In the past two decades, the narrative, in education, workplace, public services and even in sports has, in fact, swung in favour of embracing our true selves. Diversity (not just in gender) is considered a strength now. The more diverse a group is, the better is the scope for alternate opinions, ideas and styles and, therefore, the better a team performs. In many top universities, your chances of getting admitted are directly proportional to how unique your life history has been and how you can describe your special attributes. A number of organizations are punting for teams with an assortment of skills and personalities rather than standardized people. A leading IT company in artificial intelligence (AI) and the internet of things (IoT) seeks to appoint non-technical people from liberal arts backgrounds, especially with a psychology degree, to supplement the hard-wired engineers in their teams. Being yourself, pursuing your own interests, rowing your own boat or staying true are, thus, differentiating assets in this context.

So, how does one wean away from the habit of following the herd? Accepting our status, progress, achievements and unique talents is the first step. Make a list of all the achievements and talents that you think you have. Introspect if any of these came about because you tried to be someone else, and mark them in red. If your list is littered with red dots (I hope it is not), you have a lot to work on. Please note that in this exercise, we have not talked about whether your achievements and talents were appreciated by others. It's your own stocktaking. You could also surprise and impress yourself when you see the list of achievements and talents that are not marked in red. This should provide you with the conviction that you must change your behaviour to be yourself.

Now, choose a few areas where your list is marked red and your achievements are not great. These are the lowest-hanging fruits to cull out. If they didn't work out, it won't hurt to change them. Slide back to your true character. Try it a few times, at some intervals, as it takes time to perfect change. If you feel comfortable, find a partner and share your lists. Let each one of you hold the other up in this journey. The urge to deviate from the true self and behaviour will diminish gradually.

This happens at a certain point in our lives. I would like to think Life 2.0 as that moment. By then, we have accumulated enough evidence of such behaviour, anecdotes of outcomes, the wisdom to reflect on the necessity and the ability to scrutinize oneself critically. This allows the winds of change to waft in.

A cautionary tip: don't make this change of going back to being yourself because all that could be achieved by changing the behaviour has possibly been achieved and you are likely facing the law of diminishing returns. Do it only if you believe that you are better off without it, not just now, but even if the past were to be experienced again. This is not a morality dictum but a correction of something that may have happened unobtrusively.

Psychologists argue that this tendency germinates in childhood, and often, in school environments. New age parents are more sensitive to children's need to be themselves, while managing issues of their social acceptance and inclusion. Strategies to help children increase their self-worth are now built into teaching and counselling routines. This is a healthy change. It recognizes the issue and could result in future generations being less addicted to coveting alien traits. In traditional Asian schools, this transformation is yet to take roots, as children continue to be assessed through comparison.

Being ourselves is core to the concept of scripting our legacies. The story of our lives and the lessons from it flow directly from what we are and what distinctive characteristics we display. A consultant introduced me to the concept of 'table stakes' and 'differentiators' (in corporate or individual contexts). The former is what everyone has, and the latter is the special character, ability or facet that we possess and exhibit. The US has had 45 presidents so far. No one leader is spoken of as a copy of another, even though people constantly get inspired by other people who have occupied any office before them. Each leader (of the US and most other countries) was clear that his or her footsteps must be unique, historically interesting and well-remembered. The animal kingdom is the perfect example for us. Every species lives and works within its contours (and limitations), and we are fascinated by each one of them. Why did this malaise afflict the humans alone?

Artistes, musicians and sportspersons create their legacies by being unique in their styles, abilities and skills. They may reach similar outcomes and fame, but that's never because they copied another mould. Similarly, we are capable of being just us while achieving milestones and goals that we set for ourselves. The start of Life 2.0 may already be late to restore the unique self. Ideally, it should be done before significant copying or remodelling takes root.

Moderating the Ego

Swami Vivekananda (1863–1902), one of the modern spiritual thought leaders in India, said this about the ego, 'There is the mind itself. It is like a smooth lake which when struck, say by a stone, vibrates. The vibrations gather together and react on the stone, and all through the lake they will spread and be felt. The mind is like the lake; it is constantly being set in vibrations, which leave an impression on the mind; and the idea of the Ego, or personal self, the "I", is the result of these impressions. This "I" therefore is only the very rapid transmission of force and is in itself no reality.'

His analogy of the 'I' disturbing our calm minds to create the ripple of 'ego' is a simple but powerful reflection of the reality. Ego is a difficult concept to understand. Its presence is even more difficult to accept. It is perceived by others more than ourselves. Everything that we have clung on to in Life 1.0 may not have been good for us and is certainly not going to be so going forward. These could be inherent faults in our personality or acquired blemishes. We may have suffered from such infirmities or gotten away with them for the most part. Does that mean we don't need to address them at any point? Are they addressable and, even better, remediable? We will discuss the ego here, a universal problem for all, irrespective of the degree. We do not address this issue here for spiritual reformation or for cleansing the mind. That is in the realm of seekers and their gurus. Our goal here is to recognize its impact on our lives and legacy. There is never a better time to tackle the ego than when Life 2.0 begins. As always, the sooner we recognize and remedy it, the better. This is the last mandate, not because it is less important but because it is probably the most challenging of the mandates and needs a careful understanding of the concept and our degree of affliction.

Life 1.0 gives us a large set of empirical data about situations when our ego got the better of us and its consequences. The ego often colludes with, and gets aggravated by, our sense of pride, need for recognition, competitive spirit, power game, goal obsession, racing instinct, one-upmanship and, in some instances, sadistic pleasure. If we have a dominant personality, there is really no trigger required for our ego. The question is how do we still keep our pursuits without brandishing the ego? As youngsters, the ego is a signature to our profile. We let ourselves off the hook if we need to establish our supremacy in a situation. The ego drives this behaviour. We may have unleashed our ego countless times—some do it more than others. There may even be occasions when we did this subconsciously. This is even more dangerous. But people who face the consequences of their ego do take note, and some even keep mental records. A history of poor ego management is a big dent on how we are judged and, therefore, on our legacy.

Sigmund Freud propounded the three-part structure of the human psyche that encompasses the id, ego and superego.[60] He essentially distinguished between the subconscious display and the more conscious, controllable exhibition of our personas. According to Freud, the ego is the one that we can manipulate, while the other two manipulate us. This is fundamental to the understanding that some part of the ego deployment is deliberate and open to behavioural correction in us. It also confirms that an uncontrolled ego gets the better of us. So, we need to deal with it as much as we can. Thanks to Freud's categorization, we can take it up as a task.

Is there something called a 'positive ego' as some seem to believe? Pride, self-assurance, confidence, self-esteem, etc., are possible manifestations of a positive ego, and when we refer to our ego, we are generally alluding to the negative trait.

Moderation is an easier goal

One is not sure if giving up the ego totally, however desirable, is a practical goal. I certainly am nowhere near that position, and I don't want to carry the severe guilt of not achieving an unachievable goal. The more attainable goal seems to be *moderating* the ego. Moderation is possible both in quality and quantity. Reducing the number of times our ego crashes

---

[60]McLeod, Saul. 'Id, Ego, and Superego', SimplyPsychology, 2021, https://tinyurl.com/bdf7tz5f. Accessed on 4 April 2022.

through the barrier is an achievable aim. Could we also temper the scale of ego flashes? On a scale of 1–10 (10 stands for the worst form of ego manifestation), we could mitigate the number of cases that cross 5, for instance. Some baby steps towards achieving this goal can include: being defeated in a petty argument, taking a back seat in everyday family decisions like where to dine, accepting some things in life as natural like not getting tickets for a favourite show, keeping a low profile at social gatherings rather than trying to dominate them, keeping calm in airport queues, taking the service lapses of waiters in our stride, requesting for help, retaining composure when a prized thing goes missing at home, etc. I am not sure if this happens subconsciously, but I had to make an effort to implement these in my life. My wife has adopted these traits for a long time now, and it is easy for me to adopt her as a role model. I have argued with her, though, for being passive when some things happen. She, of course, has her reasons for behaving the way she does. In general, it is wise to recognize where you do not have control over things happening around you. This wisdom may come to us the hard way and rather late.

The COVID-19 pandemic rendered all of us impotent to deal with the disruption it caused in our lives, finances, relationships, and so on. It tested our calm and may have flared up our ego in frustration. Our daily lives took a different turn and we had to invent new avenues to keep our senses and priorities. In some ways, it created a conducive environment for more genuine introspection and recalibration. It may also have swung the needle of the ego decisively and even positively in many cases.

It was during the transition period of my life around 2006 that I started to read a lot of books of all kinds, besides fiction. *What Got You Here Will Not Get You Further* by Dr Marshall Goldsmith was a book that I loved reading. I could see myself in many of the situations described in the book. It was not just a wake-up call but also a point to reflect on and analyse the benefits of acting one way or another (ego-less or displaying full ego). It surely takes more time and effort to move the needle, but I began the process. It was important to realize that I did not lose anything doing so, neither financially nor in any other way. On the contrary, I started to get brownie points from my family and colleagues at work as they noticed the changes. Except for airport queues, I seem to have embraced more passivity due to which I am willing to settle for any outcome in situations where I probably sought to win earlier. That is part of the deal to moderate the ego. I am still idiosyncratic on issues like punctuality, clear communication, etc., but I am on the mend. Hopefully, at the next stage of this mandate, I would accept more shades of grey. We also have a good explanation for most such behaviours—perfectionism! However, no one is interested in the logic if the behavioural outcome is unpleasant. That takes time to sink in. The term 'trigger happy' is a good way to reinforce the need to look after the ego. Our ego spreads its wings quite a lot and can even stop us from accepting its existence! Acceptance is the starting point of dealing with it.

I had a big opportunity to dissect my ego pattern. When we co-founded an educational institution more than 14 years ago, I took on the role of steering the process before, during and after establishing the institution. However, I stayed away from putting my name on any publicity or marketing endeavours. That continues today, over 14 years later. The faces of the institution continue to be the experienced educators who are my colleagues on the board or professionals from the school leadership team. I rationalized that the satisfaction of founding and managing an educational institution, and facilitating education of large groups of youngsters, year after year, is more valuable than personal fame. It is not a major sacrifice but a small victory of sorts!

Author Todd Henry, in his popular book *Die Empty*, says, 'To countermand ego, you must adopt a posture of adaptability. This means being in a state of continual learning and openness to correction.' Learning brings enlightenment, which leads to moderating one's ego. The concept propounded by Todd Henry in this book very much resonates with the idea of Life 2.0, as his essential prescription is to complete all that you can do or give, before you die (in other words, during Life 2.0).

Often, we have the urge to change someone else's behaviour. How about doing this ourselves first?

Manifestations of the ego

As the ego itself is invisible and is a nebulous concept, we can understand its manifestations better and, simultaneously, the source of the problem. Ego and temper are synonymous in some ways. When our temper rises in a given situation, we are often not in control of our senses. This has a few consequences—arguments and unacceptable language, impolite responses, undesirable actions (including physical ones), taking on a rude tone in conversations, poor etiquette, lack of grace, breakdown of communication, snapping of relationships, undesirable body language and, overall, a bitter aftertaste and plenty of debris. If you run the event once more in your mind, you will clearly see the breaking points and the moments of madness. You will discover the more 'sober' behaviour that could have saved the day. This introspection is good because it paves the way for our internal maturity. The consequence of that maturity is the willingness to consider the ego as a problem that needs to be tackled. That is the first step to doing something with it in later life.

Readers should be able to identify with this phenomenon easily. You may have been party to one or more of the aforementioned consequences. I am told this is largely male psyche, and certainly, the males in my family are good specimens. Women seem to have a natural 'softness' in the way they respond to irritable situations. This section, then, may not be as useful to them. Many spouses may have tried and lost the battle to tame their partner's ego!

It is pertinent to note that bad ego, and its manifestations, may never be punished in the true sense and, therefore, the incentive to change has to come from within. The real punishment comes after our times, in the form of black marks on our legacy. It comes with the realization that flashing our ego may offer some task-related advantages, like getting a job done, being meticulous, etc., but it puts people off. Since people are unlikely to punish you, even if they are annoyed, you may be blissfully unaware of the worsening of your ego. Consequently, people get typecast based on their egos, and such an image and attitude becomes harder to crack. You could reflect on the friends or colleagues you have tried to avoid or taken a safe stance during your interactions with them, fearing the weight of their egos. In your minds, you have already classified such people spontaneously. Imagine if the shoe is on the other foot—you!

Ego at work, at home and in the midst of public are subtly different creatures. When our stakes are low (in a restaurant or in a commuter train, for example), we have an inversely higher propensity to display the ego (in the form of objectionable behaviour). In situations where we need to meet the same people again, the ego automatically calibrates itself. Similarly, in new situations or with new groups of people, the ego takes a relatively back seat. There are also shades of ego-led behaviour determined by hierarchy, consequences, prior encounters, potential loss or gain in stature, etc. Thus, there is an auto-valve that controls the degree of ego exhibition. If this is subconsciously possible, it raises the question: why can't we consciously self-correct our ego? After all, conscious self-correction of anything is more sustainable. For those desiring a deeper understanding of how our ego is different from our 'self', the twentieth-century Indian philosopher Ramana Maharshi[61] said, 'All bad qualities centre around the ego. When the ego is gone, "Realisation" results by itself. There are neither good nor bad qualities in the Self. The Self is free from all qualities.' So, the original stone has no defect, it has just gathered some dust.

The benefits of moderating our egos are obvious—to become a better human being, in simple language (don't we like to be called a nice person?). It also benefits our legacy by improving the way we are remembered. But, are there other advantages too? Even if the self is a different entity from the ego, it still needs the self to manage it. Psychologist Mark Leary has pointed out in his book *The Curse of the Self* that while the self can be our greatest resource, it can also be our darkest enemy. The self has a self-serving goal. This goal comes in the way of us seeking humility, acceptance and gentle behaviour that are unquestioned virtues. Tempering the ego is a first step towards such higher-order human behaviour. As the researchers Jack Bauer, Heidi Wayment, and Kateryna Sylaska put it, 'The volume of the ego is turned down so that it might listen to others as well as

---

[61]Sri Ramana Maharshi, https://tinyurl.com/2p8a35zz. Accessed on 4 April 2022.

the self in an effort to approach life more humanely and compassionately.[62] The term they coined in their paper—the 'quiet ego'—is an acceptance of the trait but with a muted manifestation. Here again, they allude to moderating the ego rather than the more onerous task of eliminating it. There are no monetary or other rewards in this pursuit. However, it does have indirect health benefits of stabilizing our blood pressure and maintaining our mental balance, which arises from behaviours that are moderated. Another more distant benefit is that we may become more likeable, which stems from a lowered ego. Psychometric tests are part of corporate recruitment and often include test for a dominant ego. The world is becoming one big, connected 'people's place' where human interactions are said to determine our progress—individually and collectively. Anything that comes in the way of healthy collaboration, like the ego, are frowned upon and can be disqualifiers.

Why should this be attempted in Life 2.0? It could be done earlier for sure. It could be argued that for behaviour change, a few things are mandatory. There must be a reflective process, the experience of aberration and anecdotal triggers, an acceptance of the need for change, a commitment to change and a method to monitor the progress of change. It, therefore, requires a certain level of

---

[62]Wayment, Heidi, Jack Bauer and Kateryna Sylaska. 'The Quiet Ego Scale: Measuring the Compassionate Self-Identity', *Journal of Happiness Studies*, Vol. 16, 2015, 999-1033, https://tinyurl.com/yckncfcr. Accessed on 4 April 2022.

maturity and freedom from incentives like money, power, etc. At the crossroads for Life 2.0, it is expected that we would have transcended these incentives and provocations. We are, therefore, willing to sit down with ourselves and critically evaluate our flaws and behaviours. Those of us who develop this ability will see the advantages of seeking that change. Our reflection may also be triggered by our experiences (getting turned down for several jobs or not being able to build durable social assets, for instance), and by observing the behaviours of others around us that may seem different, and more desirable than ours.

What can help this process of reformation? Failures and controversies do, but we don't have to break eggs, if we don't need to. Here are some simple recommendations to achieve this transformation:

- Slowing down our responses
- Pausing (or even postponing) any riposte
- Not participating in some arguments
- Picking our battles wisely (maybe the more important ones)
- Venting privately
- Sleeping over an issue
- Focusing on the issue rather than the person involved
- Meditating
- Having an ombudsman to watch your behaviour (and give feedback)
- Being gracious to the other person involved in the scene

THE MANDATES: COORDINATES OF A NEW JOURNEY

- Writing a diary note instead of a verbal response
- Writing is often a good restorative therapy for anger and annoyance.

Some of these are easy to practice, while the others are hardwired in us. Tapping into a personal coach is another effective way to start addressing a stubborn habit. As a first step, do a secret poll among your immediate colleagues, family or friends on your ability to manage your ego. Ask them to respond to a few simple questions on a scale of 1 to 5 (5 representing the best behaviour). If you are good at receiving feedback, you will appreciate it and act on the results straightaway. Although, your ego may refuse to accept the results! Unlike some of the other areas of transformation in this book, moderating our ego is generally reversible (you can quickly go back to the old bad habit). Thus, you must build in disincentives for slipping back. The best way is to also have someone monitor your progress, alert you about any slippage and urge better compliance. Become a mentee. There are interesting parallels to be drawn here with the rehabilitation process for alcoholics and even convicts because the ego may also be an addiction.

THE STORY OF HOW MY LIFE 2.0 BEGAN...

Coincidentally or otherwise, the tipping point for embracing the 12 mandates in this book occurred to me around the same time in 2006. I am thankful for that stroke of fate. In this concluding chapter, I am allowing myself the indulgence of narrating the sequence of how I set foot in my Life 2.0.

A short account of some incidents leading up to this moment could be useful to understand my frame of mind that was formed largely in my younger years. When I was deciding my field of college education, I was caught between a strong family current towards studying engineering and my own preference for an accounting career. Both my brothers pursued engineering degrees. I must have ruffled quite a few feathers at home when I fought the tide. It taught me two things—I must exercise my mind whenever the need arises, and I need to figure out where my natural interests lie. People who believe that they did not pursue the education that they would have liked to would empathize with these

THE STORY OF HOW MY LIFE 2.0 BEGAN...

thoughts. Many engineers of my generation gave up on the subject completely and ended up in totally unrelated fields like brand marketing or banking—electrical engineers who manage 'current' accounts is a funny quip I have heard! It was also implicit that I took complete responsibility for my choices.

The next twist was when I was choosing my first job after acquiring a management degree. The general tendency was towards the more famous multinational companies like Unilever, Procter & Gamble (P&G), Citibank, Bank of America, etc. The money and the glamour were too tempting, although those were not the only talking points. I had to choose between P&G (Richardson Hindustan at that time) and Tube Investments, Chennai. The latter was a staid South Indian group back then, which was trying to bring in management graduates. They were recruiting from campus for the first time. As it turned out, my Tube Investments experience was great and my learning went up several notches. Seven of us joined the company at that time from the same business school, and all of us have had stellar careers since then. I can't quite claim that I knew this all along, but I was willing to give my instincts a chance. The good thing about a career (as opposed to other life decisions) is that you can always retract and redirect yourself quickly if your previous choice doesn't feel right (see the section on reassessing goals, page 49).

There were further twists in my life, some natural and others self-made. Six years into my first career in accounting,

I felt saturated and was looking for a change. A commercial role that progressed into a full-fledged sales job came my way. I lapped it up, even though my sales and people skills had not been established or tested. But it seemed to fit my passion better. It turned out to be a game changer for me, as I have since been a sales and marketing professional! With such career moves, I guess I developed an intuitive sense of preparedness for change—gradual as well as disruptive. My adaptive skill became my core competence, if you will. This helped me immensely when the moment of Life 2.0 arrived.

How dramatically 2006 unfolded for me!

That year brought in a sudden turn of events in my life—there was a huge churn. The list runs like this: the loss of a well-paying, satisfying job (which I had held for about 15 years), the loss of a dear relative (and a father figure), an unexciting start to a new consulting venture, alarming trends towards a physical disability that I had been diagnosed with, career insecurity and a kiss of death (yes, I survived by maybe 120 seconds). This period of six months caused an unprecedented amount of uncertainty in my life. Seconds seemed like minutes, minutes like hours and a month took forever to pass. It also coincided with my mid-life, and the idea of a potential crisis kept haunting me.

In early 2006, I returned to Singapore, after a year-long stint in the US, to my old job in the same company. A new global leader had taken over the top job and was making changes. The company, a private equity-owned enterprise, was gearing up to announce its Initial Public Offering (IPO).

The focus was on cost-cutting and, hence, over a hundred people across the organization were let go and teams were restructured. My boss, who had helmed the Asia operation for about 16 years, was given the notice first. I was, in some ways, positioned to succeed him, but a German confidante (the company was German-owned and largely run by Germans) was brought in. In the restructuring that continued, I lost my job. Given that I had a strong record in the company over the years, this was a disappointing end, but that is the corporate reality. With a limited severance package and an uncertain future, I started on the long road to re-employment. I was perhaps unprepared for this too, even though I could see the constant tinkering of leadership positions in the company. This phenomenon happens in multinational companies quite regularly, but when it hits you, the first experience is not nice.

I still continued with the plans to go on vacation to India for about 15 days, one of our first long, multi-city family vacations. From Chennai to Kochi to Trivandrum to Nagercoil to Thiruchendur to Madurai to Trichy and all places in between in South India, we were on the road, enjoying beaches, hotels, temples everywhere, and it was great fun. It was clearly the best antidote to my situation then. There is no better way to bond as a family than travelling together. It was a double delight as our daughter was approaching her senior years at school, and we reckoned it was our one last chance to do such a long trip with her.

The initial distress gave way to an awakening of my independent spirits. I was not keen to start a new job and wanted to try my hand at my own consulting or training stint. There was some sense of financial sufficiency though. A couple of months went by in resizing my mind and crystallizing options. Our daughter had two more years to go at high school and, hence, a steady income was important and so was the location. Soon after this, I lost my grandfather. Even though he was 93 and had lived a full life, I felt quite orphaned. For over 40 years, he was my best family companion, and I had always looked up to him for inspiration for the way he singularly shaped his somewhat meaningless existence as a retired civil servant into being a reputed music critic and a revered writer. He was the perfect example of a life-long learner and had reformatted his life a few times. He was also a role model for frugality, sociability and contentment. He passed away after a very brief illness, but it was unexpected. It took me more time to adjust to his loss than my own job loss.

Subsequently, I opened a consulting company and started to tap into my contacts for early meetings with potential clients. Perhaps I was not approaching it correctly, and success was elusive. In the meantime, my wife and I had one of those meditative chats and allowed our minds to imagine the possibilities without restraint. The thought of doing our own business kept coming back in our conversations. Some ideas presented a smaller prospect than others, and some appeared to be commodity businesses.

Finally, we narrowed our options down to education. I had worked in many entrepreneurial environments, and this spirit had been infused in me along with the thought process to overcome a risk-averse mindset.

During this period, with little new income coming in, my wife and I were so focused on the next big thing that we had no time or inclination to brood over the present. This was our greatest achievement, in hindsight. Our energy was spent fully on creating our future. We did not wallow in self-pity or go on ruminating. I was also not quite resentful at the turn of events and looked upon the situation as an opportunity to reboot. The fact that my wife and I shared a similar attitude to money, lifestyle and comfort helped a lot. The next project that could use our experiences and abilities was almost taking shape.

Two other significant developments shook my life around the same time. I was swimming alone in my apartment complex pool on a December evening, also in 2006! Due to the holidays, the pool was empty. I was an occasional swimmer with limited skills. Either due to my limited skills, fatigue, cramps or a combination of all three, I started going down to the bottom after swimming for about half an hour. Luckily, I had the presence of mind to shout for help and raise my hands a couple of times above water. My wife had been away at a store all this while. My sister-in-law who was passing by with her young daughter fortuitously noticed my cries and alerted some people nearby. I was lucky again, as one of the two people she approached in the complex near the pool was a swimmer. He jumped in and pulled me out. Fortunately, he also had the skills to quickly resuscitate me. By the time my wife arrived at the scene, I was out of the water, breathing and waiting for an ambulance. I was half-conscious and was asked to answer simple questions to keep my systems active. I reckon everything happened in the nick of time—perhaps 120 seconds later, it could have ended quite differently. God had played his part through my sister-in-law and an unknown soul. Their rescue act was far above any gratitude that I could offer. I reached out to my saviour and wrote him a mail thanking him, with an invitation to join me for tea. The young man was embarrassed and told me that he only did what anyone in his position would have done and politely bowed out of my tea invite. You can easily mark this as a moment of second life. This moment also had a lesson about helping others without fanfare or without expecting any rewards, and it was taught by a gem of a youngster.

As if such drama was not enough, I had also been diagnosed with a debilitating disease that would gradually cripple my functionality. The clock was ticking, and no treatment has been found for this disease yet. It has been a 15-year regression, and could leave me with about five to eight more years of reasonable functionality. This diagnosis also brought in an important perspective to the way I had to imagine my future. It meant, in some way, that I had to fast-track the fulfilment of my new goals. I wasn't prepared to shrink my goals. What I wanted to do with my life had, thus, acquired a vastly different dimension and time frame.

This is where the notion of Life 2.0 began for me, with a lot of unexpected drama, churn, disruption and urge to reboot.

So what heralded my 2.0 life? My wife and I decided to relaunch ourselves professionally. We considered setting up a school. One thing was clear to us. It had to be a high-quality institution with a strong brand power. Many years of corporate life had taught me the virtues of a joint venture. One of the groups I had worked with for several years had more than 10 successful joint ventures in many new fields that were unfamiliar to the group. This was achieved by partnering with people or companies who were experts. We found an education partner who had the necessary expertise and values similar to ours. No one in our immediate families had experience with running a business, and the only familiar grounds for us were honesty, hard work, quality and trust. The will was there, but the way had to be found. We did not have to wait for long, and the project blossomed rapidly. Fifteen months after my phone call with the promoters, the school began. Along the way, I learnt a lot of lessons about life, some of which are reflected in this book.

While the school project was taking shape, I was fortunate enough to get into another activity that I was interested in—teaching. Thanks to my brother's introduction, I started teaching at two prestigious universities in Singapore. I sought and introduced my pet subject of sales management into their curricula, with a syllabus that I designed. My teaching stint lasted for about a decade and led me into executive education, another natural extension of university teaching. All these were very different activities compared to my corporate life of 25 years. In many ways, my rediscovery was fully on its way, and so was Life 2.0.

I was fortunate to find my voice through writing and added that to my vocational list (of Life 2.0). Writing had always been interesting for me, but writing books professionally looked like a tall order. My first experiments with writing articles for a leading business newspaper went well and stimulated me more. It still took a few years before I could see a big outcome. My first book on account management was published by Palgrave Macmillan in May 2018, and the next one on habits for skill-building by Penguin in 2021. I am hopeful that I can write more in the future. This life-transforming journey has given me the context, time, reflective mindset and the awakening to embrace many of the guiding postulates that I have articulated in this book. Thus, Life 2.0 has clearly been a gainful reboot for me.

The satisfying part of all this is that most of these activities have happened internally. This is important for aiming at the higher levels of self-attainment that Abraham Maslow theorized. I am confident that readers will have the same thoughts and stimulus that I had while embarking on these changes.

Here, an important question needs to be answered—how much of the new path was initiated and how much was accidental? As most would guess, it was a mix, but I would like to imagine that many of the triggers were unplanned. Starting a school or writing a book cannot be accidents, but the genesis can be! Did I receive a fortuitous opportunity to begin Life 2.0 and start rescripting my life? Absolutely so! I have shared examples from my own life merely as a peer (and to offer hope to everyone!). The fact that I was not afraid of change even in Life 1.0 did help. Life 2.0 does dawn at some point, often linked to some events in life. That is the moment for all new things.

THE BEGINNING

I would call this the 'beginning' for many readers like you rather than the conclusion of this book. The beginning of a new and more mindful regime. The 12 mandates in this book perhaps beckon as much to you as they did to me at various points in time. The circumstances that trigger your Life 2.0 would certainly be different from mine, but if you reckon that they are hovering around you, and are seemingly different from the past, this is the time to reflect and reimagine life. As Life 2.0 starts to unfold in front of you, it commands you to take control in ways that you have always liked to.

What I have realized is that there is a midway point between being an ascetic and a materialist, and that is a very large viable space. It suits many of us. It does not call for renouncing everything and turning fully spiritual, but it allows for living a mainstream life with some changes to our activities, thoughts, goals and behaviours. It can run parallel to a normal life, with a few adjustments. This is not a change of car or an overhaul. It's just upgrading its functioning. In the process, you come to recognize your blind spots and acquire the necessary tools to deal with them.

You don't need to do it as haphazardly as I did, sometimes unaware of setting off on a new journey. Hopefully, you see this book as a guide for your reboot and a successful journey to a good legacy. You must be cognizant of your uniqueness and be willing to be unconventional or even counterintuitive. The past is not really the pattern you may want in the future. You probably may even discover other elements of the script that I did not encounter. Apart from time and inclination, no other resources are necessary for this journey, so it is economical as well! It allows for gentle starts and multiple attempts as long as you maintain a set of ultimate goals and push yourself towards them with determination. What's more, we are the sole judge of our results! There is greatness in everyone, only if we unearth it. If we let the Life 2.0 opportunity go by, that greatness remains bottled and leaves with us when we leave the world. Please remember: we are only what we choose to do. When we travel this road, we are all novices. As the nineteenth-century American artist Ralph Waldo Emerson said, 'Every artist is first an amateur.' However, we will progress to the legacy goals very quickly as we stay on course in our Life 2.0. Take yourself on! Develop your script with you as the central character and start a new life—Life 2.0.

I am happy to receive comments or allied ideas and experiences from you. Please email me at shankar.bala.s@gmail.com.

ACKNOWLEDGEMENTS

I am not very clear about what came first: writing this book or chronicling the episodes in the lives of the many people I know or have read about. As the topic of what constitutes shaping an interesting legacy germinated in my thoughts, I reached out to more people who, in my reckoning, had carried themselves smartly and consciously to the tree that will bear them the fruit of legacy. I sincerely thank the several friends and colleagues whose fascinating and powerful stories form an integral part of this book, as much as the anecdotes of famous personalities.

My very special thanks are due to the legendary cricketer Anil Kumble for readily agreeing to write a foreword for the book. I couldn't have gotten a better person for doing the honours. Kumble is a hugely respected person not only for his cricketing exploits but also for his urbane and dignified character. He wears all these with consummate ease. His is a rare breed in the world of competitive sports.

Dr Bindu Hari, of the NPS group of schools, and my friend S. S. Rasaily, of Vidyatech, extended support in critical ways when I asked them to. Endorsements are important for any book, especially from those who have top credentials in their personal or professional lives or both. The people who I reached out to have achieved trailblazing feats in many ways. A big thanks to Dr M.B. Athreya, Mr R.S. Pawar, Ms Rama Bijapurkar, Professor Raj Srivastava and Ms Meena Ganesh.

Families often play selfless roles while writing books. I must thank my inner circle—my wife, Alamelu, and my daughter, Rashmi—they have been my unpaid editors, proofreaders, critics, artists and sounding boards for ideas. I often had to raise my game to secure their approval. My mother, Rajalakshmi, is among the few people I know who is ever ready to change, which I find endlessly inspiring, especially for a topic such as this one. She decoupled her life from finances about six decades ago!

Finally, I thank my publishers, especially Yamini Chowdhury, Saswati Bora, Sneha Bhagwat and the Rupa team for seeing early merit in this theme and for painstakingly and patiently guiding this book till it reached your hands, despite the uncertainty and delays posed by the pandemic.